28 Days to a Lighter You

Somatic Yoga Weight Loss Challenge

Helen Talbott

Copyright Page

Disclaimer

The information contained in this book, 28 Days to a Lighter You: Somatic Yoga Weight Loss Challenge, is provided for informational purposes only and is not intended to be a substitute for professional medical advice, diagnosis, or treatment.

While the author has taken reasonable precautions to ensure the accuracy of the information contained herein, no warranty, express or implied, is made as to the accuracy, completeness, or reliability of the information provided. You should not rely on any information contained in this book as a substitute for professional medical advice from a qualified healthcare provider.

Always seek the advice of your physician or other qualified healthcare professional with any questions you may have regarding a medical condition. Never disregard professional medical advice or delay in seeking it because of something you have read in this book.

The author and publisher disclaim any liability or responsibility for any harm or injury resulting directly or indirectly from the use and application of any of the contents of this book. If you are pregnant, nursing, or have any pre-existing medical conditions, it is strongly recommended that you consult with your healthcare provider before undertaking any new exercise or wellness program.

Please note that individual results may vary, and weight loss is influenced by a variety of factors beyond the scope of this book.

By using this book, you acknowledge and agree to the terms of this disclaimer.

Table of contents

About the Author

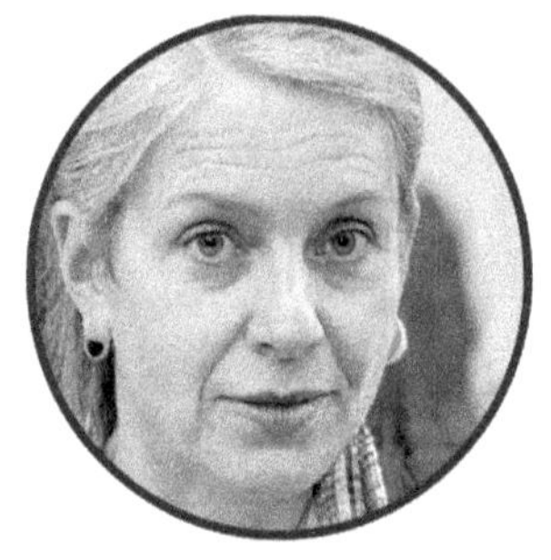

Hello, lovely souls! I'm Helen Talbott, your guide on this transformative journey towards a lighter, healthier version of yourself. As a certified yoga instructor and holistic wellness coach, I've witnessed firsthand the incredible power of somatic yoga in facilitating weight loss and fostering a deeper mind-body connection. Through this 28-day challenge, I'm thrilled to share with you a carefully curated blend of yoga poses, mindful eating practices, and self-care rituals designed to help you shed physical weight while also shedding emotional baggage. My passion for helping others discover their true potential fuels every word on these pages, and I invite you to join me as we embark on this empowering adventure together. Remember, each day is an opportunity for growth and renewal, and I'm here to support you every step of the way. Let's dive in and embrace the journey towards a lighter, brighter you! With love and light, Helen Talbott

Introduction

Welcome to the Journey: What is Somatic Yoga and How Can it Help You Lose Weight?

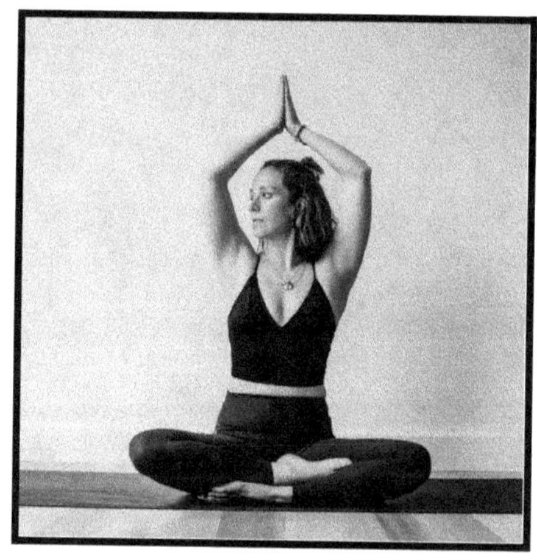

Embrace a transformation beyond the physical with Somatic Yoga! This 28-day challenge invites you to discover a mindful movement practice that goes beyond calorie burning and unlocks sustainable weight loss by addressing the whole you: body, mind, and spirit.

So, what is Somatic Yoga? Unlike traditional yoga styles that focus on external alignment, Somatic Yoga dives inward. It invites you to explore your body's sensations, rediscover its natural movement patterns, and cultivate a deep sense of embodied awareness. Instead of pushing into challenging poses, we'll explore gentle movements and guided explorations, gently coaxing your body to release tension, improve flexibility, and rediscover its optimal alignment.

But how can this lead to weight loss? Here's the magic:

- **Mindful Movement:** By listening to your body's needs and respecting its limitations, you'll avoid injuries and build sustainable exercise habits.

- **Stress Reduction:** Chronic stress hinders weight loss. Somatic Yoga's calming practices decrease cortisol levels, promoting deeper sleep and a calmer mind, both crucial for healthy weight management.
- **Improved Body Awareness:** When you're truly in tune with your body, you can make mindful choices about food and movement, avoiding restrictive diets and embracing intuitive eating.
- **Increased Metabolism:** Gentle movements activate different muscle groups, boosting your metabolism and helping your body burn more calories throughout the day.
- **Holistic Transformation:** Somatic Yoga not only addresses the physical but also cultivates self-compassion and

mindful eating habits, creating a lasting foundation for a healthier lifestyle.

This 28-day journey will guide you through a progressive series of Somatic Yoga practices, breathwork exercises, and mindful reflections. As you connect with your body and unlock its innate wisdom, you'll not only experience weight loss but also cultivate a more balanced, stress-free, and empowered you.

Are you ready to embark on this transformative journey? Let's begin!

Setting Your Intentions: Defining Your Goals and Creating a Supportive Mindset

Welcome to Day 2 of your 28-day Somatic Yoga Weight Loss Challenge! Today, we dive deep into **setting your intentions**, a crucial step for a successful and fulfilling journey.

Defining Your Goals:

- **Go beyond "weight loss":** While shedding pounds is a common desire, explore its deeper motivations. Do you want increased energy, improved health, or more confidence? Aligning your goals with your "why" fosters long-term commitment.
- Make it **SMART**: Specific, Measurable, Achievable, Relevant, and Time-bound. Instead of "get healthier," try "complete 20 minutes of somatic yoga practice 3 times a week."
- **Focus on progress, not perfection:** Set realistic, achievable goals.

Celebrate small wins and remember, setbacks are part of the process.

Cultivating a Supportive Mindset:

- **Shift the focus from deprivation to abundance:** View Somatic Yoga as an enriching gift to your body and mind, not a punishment.
- **Embrace self-compassion:** Be kind to yourself, especially during challenging moments. Acknowledge your strengths and celebrate your progress.
- **Visualize success:** Imagine yourself achieving your goals and feeling the positive emotions associated with them. This empowers your journey.
- **Find your support system:** Share your goals with loved ones, join online communities, or seek professional guidance for ongoing motivation.

Activities:

- **Journaling:** Write down your weight loss goals, deeper motivations, and desired health outcomes. Reflect on your current mindset and areas for improvement.
- **Vision board:** Create a visual representation of your goals, including images, affirmations, and inspiring quotes. Visualize this board daily to stay motivated.
- **Affirmations:** Repeat positive statements about yourself and your journey, like "I am worthy of health and well-being" or "I am committed to taking care of myself."

Remember, setting intentions is an ongoing process. Revisit your goals and mindset regularly, adapt as needed, and most importantly, trust your journey! Let's move forward with clarity, compassion, and a supportive mindset for a transformative experience.

Ready to step into your lighter, healthier self? Let's do this!

Essential Somatic Yoga Principles for Weight Loss:

Somatic Yoga offers a unique approach to weight loss, focusing on cultivating mindful movement, body awareness, and holistic well-being. Here are some core principles that set it apart from traditional exercise regimes and contribute to sustainable weight management:

1. Embodied Awareness:

- **Tune into internal sensations:** Instead of solely focusing on external form, Somatic Yoga encourages you to listen to your body's signals about tension, comfort, and range of motion. This awareness helps you adjust poses intuitively, avoiding forced alignment and potential injuries.
- **Explore gentle movements:** Gentle explorations and micro-movements activate smaller muscle groups and

fascia, aiding in releasing chronic tension and improving proprioception (body awareness). This subtle activation can improve metabolism and energy expenditure throughout the day.

2. Breathwork & Nervous System Regulation:

- **Conscious breathing:** Somatic Yoga practices incorporate mindful breathing techniques, promoting relaxation and calming the nervous system. This helps combat stress, a major contributor to weight gain, by lowering cortisol levels and fostering restful sleep.
- **Somatic nervous system regulation:** Through gentle movements and breathwork, Somatic Yoga can help activate the parasympathetic nervous system (rest and digest), promoting better digestion and nutrient absorption.

3. Mindful Eating & Intuitive Choices:

- **Connect with food cravings:** Somatic Yoga cultivates a mindful relationship with food by encouraging awareness of physical and emotional hunger cues. This helps you distinguish true hunger from emotional eating and make conscious choices about food.
- **Develop intuitive eating:** By listening to your body's needs and responding to its signals, you can naturally gravitate towards nourishing foods and healthy portion sizes. This fosters a sustainable approach to eating without restrictive diets.

4. Sustainable Movement Habits:

- **Find joy in movement:** Somatic Yoga focuses on cultivating a positive relationship with movement. Gentle explorations and personalized practices foster joy and intrinsic motivation, encouraging you to integrate movement into your daily life beyond structured workouts.

- **Listen to your body:** Somatic Yoga emphasizes honoring your body's needs and avoiding pushing into pain. This prevents injuries and fosters a sustainable practice you can enjoy for life.

Remember:

- **Holistic approach:** Somatic Yoga addresses weight loss beyond the physical, promoting mental and emotional well-being for a lasting transformation.
- **Individualized practice:** Each body is unique. Adapt poses to your needs and avoid comparing yourself to others.
- **Consistency is key:** Regular practice is more important than intensity. Start

with shorter sessions and gradually increase duration as you progress.

By embracing these principles, you can embark on a transformative journey with Somatic Yoga, experiencing sustainable weight loss while fostering a deeper connection with your body and mind.

Chapter 1

Week 1: Foundations of Somatic Movement

Welcome to the first week of your 28-Day Somatic Yoga Weight Loss Challenge! This week focuses on establishing the fundamentals of mindful movement and body awareness, the cornerstones of your transformative journey.

Day 1: Embodiment & Awareness - Tuning into Your Body's Signals

Our adventure begins with cultivating **embodied awareness**, learning to listen to your body's subtle messages. Start by finding a quiet space and lying down comfortably. Close your eyes and take a few deep breaths, allowing your body to settle.

- **Body Scan:** Gently focus your attention on different parts of your body, starting with your toes and slowly moving upwards. Notice any sensations of tension, pressure, or discomfort. Simply observe without judgment.

- **Gentle Stretches:** Perform gentle stretches for your neck, shoulders, and arms, paying attention to how your body responds to each movement. Avoid pushing into pain; prioritize comfort and ease.

Day 2: Breathwork & Relaxation - Unwinding Tension and Calming the Mind

Breathwork plays a crucial role in Somatic Yoga, influencing nervous system regulation and relaxation. Today, we explore two calming breath practices:

- **Diaphragmatic Breathing:** Lie down comfortably and place one hand on your belly and the other on your chest. As you inhale, feel your belly expand, pushing your hand outwards. Exhale slowly, drawing your belly button inwards. Repeat for several minutes, focusing on deep, smooth breaths.

- **Alternate Nostril Breathing:** Sit comfortably with your spine erect. Close your right nostril with your thumb and inhale deeply through your left nostril. Close your left nostril with your ring finger and exhale slowly through your right nostril. Repeat by inhaling through your right nostril and exhaling through your left. Continue for several minutes.

Day 3: Gentle Movement & Exploration - Discovering Your Range of Motion

Today, we move gently, exploring your body's natural range of motion without forcing poses. Remember, prioritize comfort and listen to your body's signals.

- **Neck Rolls:** Slowly roll your head in a circular motion, first clockwise and then counterclockwise. Avoid any sharp movements or discomfort.

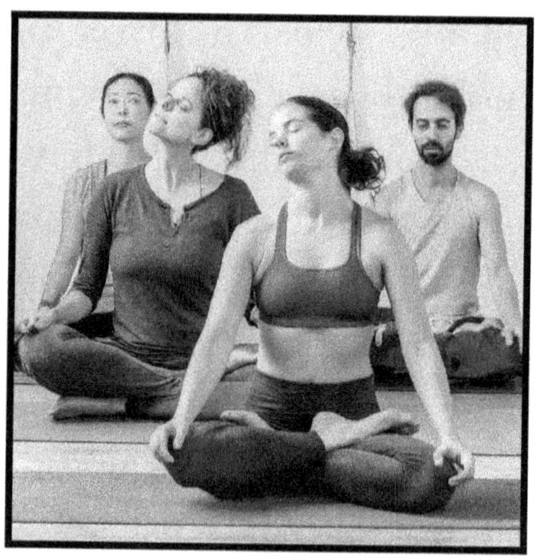

- **Shoulder Shrugs:** Gently shrug your shoulders up towards your ears and then relax them down. Repeat a few times, observing how your neck and chest respond.

- **Arm Circles:** Make small circles with your arms, forward and backward. Gradually increase the size of the circles as your body feels comfortable.

Day 4: Somatic Practices for Digestion & Metabolism

Gentle movements can positively impact digestion and metabolism. Here are two simple practices to explore:

- **Seated Spinal Twists:** Sit comfortably with your legs crossed or extended in front of you. Gently twist your upper body to one side, placing your hand on your opposite knee for support. Hold for a few breaths and repeat on the other side.

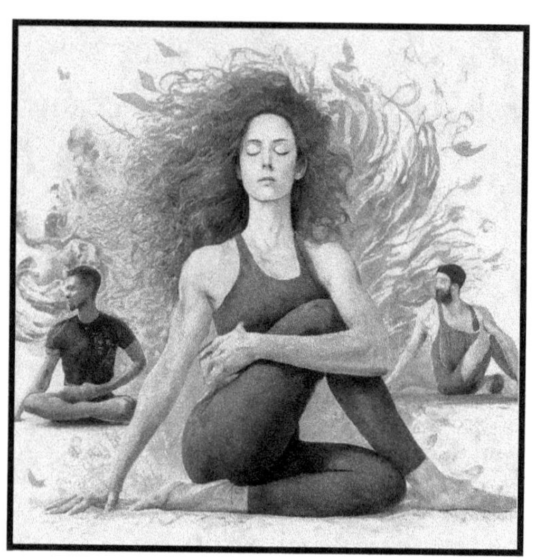

- **Knee Hugs:** Lie down on your back and bring one knee towards your chest, hugging it with both arms. Hold for a few breaths and repeat with the other leg.

Day 5: Rest & Reflection - Integrating New Awareness and Practices

Take some time today to reflect on your journey so far. Write down your experiences, challenges, and insights gained. Remember, progress takes time and consistency. Be kind to yourself and celebrate your efforts!

Bonus Tip: As you move throughout your day, bring your awareness to your breath and body sensations. This mindful approach helps you stay connected to your inner wisdom and make conscious choices.

Remember, this is just the beginning of your Somatic Yoga adventure. Stay tuned for week 2, where we'll delve deeper into building your Somatic Flow!

Chapter 2

Week 2: Building Your Somatic Flow

Day 1: Embodiment & Awareness - Tuning into Your Body's Signals

Welcome to Day 1 of your Somatic Yoga Weight Loss Challenge! Today, we embark on a journey inward, cultivating **embodied awareness**, the foundation of your transformative experience. Remember, this is not about achieving perfect poses, but about connecting with your body's unique needs and respecting its wisdom.

Setting the Stage:

- **Find a quiet space:** Eliminate distractions and create an environment where you can fully focus on yourself.

- **Prepare your body:** Wear comfortable clothing that allows for gentle movement. You can practice on a yoga mat, blanket, or even your bed.
- **Begin with stillness:** Lie down comfortably on your back or your side, whichever feels more supportive. Close your eyes or soften your gaze downwards.

Body Scan:

- **Start with your toes:** Gently bring your attention to your right foot, noticing any sensations of warmth, coolness, pressure, or tingling. Simply observe without judgment.
- **Travel upwards:** Gradually move your awareness up your leg, noticing subtle sensations in your ankles, calves, and thighs. Do the same for your left leg.
- **Explore your core:** Pay attention to your abdomen, pelvis, and lower back.

Are there any areas of tension or tightness? Observe without judgment.

- **Move to your torso:** Scan your chest, ribs, and shoulders. Notice any areas holding onto breath or tension.
- **Neck and head:** Gently bring your awareness to your neck, jaw, and head. Are there any areas of tightness or discomfort?
- **Return to stillness:** Take a few deep breaths, allowing your body to settle. Notice how you feel overall.

Gentle Stretches:

- **Neck rolls:** Slowly roll your head in a circular motion, first clockwise and then counterclockwise, staying within a comfortable range. Avoid any sharp movements or discomfort.
- **Shoulder shrugs:** Gently shrug your shoulders up towards your ears and then relax them down. Repeat a few

times, observing how your neck and chest respond.

- **Arm circles:** Make small circles with your arms, forward and backward. Gradually increase the size of the circles as your body feels comfortable.

Journaling:

- Take a few minutes to write down your experiences from today's practice. What sensations did you notice in your body? Were there any areas of tension or discomfort? How did you feel overall?
- Write down a personal commitment for incorporating more mindful awareness into your day. Choose something small and achievable, like taking mindful breaths throughout the day or paying attention to how your body feels when you sit or walk.

Remember:

- This is a starting point, not a destination. Be patient with yourself and explore at your own pace.
- There is no right or wrong way to experience this practice. Trust your body's wisdom and listen to its signals.
- Every moment is an opportunity to cultivate embodiment. As you move throughout your day, bring your awareness to your breath and body sensations.

Enjoy the journey towards a mindful and embodied you!

Day 2: Breathwork & Relaxation - Unwinding Tension and Calming the Mind

Welcome to Day 2 of your Somatic Yoga Weight Loss Challenge! Today, we delve into the calming world of **breathwork**, exploring practices to soothe your nervous system and release tension. Remember, consistent practice is key, so even a few minutes of dedicated breathing can make a difference.

Setting the Stage:

- **Prepare your space:** Find a quiet, comfortable area where you can sit or lie down without distractions. You can use a yoga mat, blanket, or even your bed.
- **Settle your body:** Choose a position that feels supportive, either lying on your back, sitting upright with your spine tall, or sitting cross-legged. Close

your eyes or soften your gaze downwards.

- **Find your anchor:** Place one hand on your belly and the other on your chest. This helps you focus on the movement of your breath.

Diaphragmatic Breathing:

- Imagine your belly as a balloon. As you inhale slowly through your nose, feel your belly expand, pushing your hand outwards.
- Exhale slowly through your mouth, allowing your belly to gently deflate, like the air leaving the balloon.
- Focus on the natural rise and fall of your abdomen with each breath. Don't force anything, simply observe the flow.
- Practice for 5-10 minutes, noticing how your body relaxes with each breath.

Alternate Nostril Breathing:

- Sit comfortably with your spine erect. Close your right nostril with your thumb and inhale deeply through your left nostril.
- Close your left nostril with your ring finger and exhale slowly through your right nostril.
- Repeat by inhaling through your right nostril and exhaling through your left.
- Continue this pattern for 5-7 minutes, focusing on the calming rhythm of your breath.

Deepening Relaxation:

- After your breathwork, spend a few minutes in quiet reflection. Observe any changes in your body, mind, and emotions.
- You can gently scan your body for any remaining tension and release it with a deep exhale.

- Visualize yourself surrounded by calmness and peace.

Journaling:

- Reflect on your experience with today's practices. Which one did you find more calming? Did you notice any physical or mental shifts?
- Write down a personal intention for incorporating more breathwork into your daily life. Could you practice a few minutes of mindful breathing in the morning, during stressful moments, or before sleep?

Remember:

- Breathwork is a personal journey. Experiment with different techniques and find what works best for you.
- Consistency is key. Even short, regular breathwork sessions can bring significant benefits.

- Be patient and kind to yourself. Learning to calm your mind and body takes time and practice.

Enjoy the process of unwinding tension and cultivating inner peace with every breath!

Day 2: Breathwork & Relaxation - Unwinding Tension and Calming the Mind

Welcome to Day 2 of your Somatic Yoga Weight Loss Challenge! Today, we delve into the calming world of **breathwork**, exploring practices to soothe your nervous system and release tension. Remember, consistent practice is key, so even a few minutes of dedicated breathing can make a difference.

Setting the Stage:

- **Prepare your space:** Find a quiet, comfortable area where you can sit or lie down without distractions. You can use a yoga mat, blanket, or even your bed.
- **Settle your body:** Choose a position that feels supportive, either lying on your back, sitting upright with your spine tall, or sitting cross-legged. Close your eyes or soften your gaze downwards.

- **Find your anchor:** Place one hand on your belly and the other on your chest. This helps you focus on the movement of your breath.

Diaphragmatic Breathing:

- Imagine your belly as a balloon. As you inhale slowly through your nose, feel your belly expand, pushing your hand outwards.
- Exhale slowly through your mouth, allowing your belly to gently deflate, like the air leaving the balloon.
- Focus on the natural rise and fall of your abdomen with cach brcath. Don't force anything, simply observe the flow.
- Practice for 5-10 minutes, noticing how your body relaxes with each breath.

Alternate Nostril Breathing:

- Sit comfortably with your spine erect. Close your right nostril with your thumb and inhale deeply through your left nostril.
- Close your left nostril with your ring finger and exhale slowly through your right nostril.
- Repeat by inhaling through your right nostril and exhaling through your left.
- Continue this pattern for 5-7 minutes, focusing on the calming rhythm of your breath.

Deepening Relaxation:

- After your breathwork, spend a few minutes in quiet reflection. Observe any changes in your body, mind, and emotions.
- You can gently scan your body for any remaining tension and release it with a deep exhale.

- Visualize yourself surrounded by calmness and peace.

Journaling:

- Reflect on your experience with today's practices. Which one did you find more calming? Did you notice any physical or mental shifts?
- Write down a personal intention for incorporating more breathwork into your daily life. Could you practice a few minutes of mindful breathing in the morning, during stressful moments, or before sleep?

Remember:

- Breathwork is a personal journey. Experiment with different techniques and find what works best for you.
- Consistency is key. Even short, regular breathwork sessions can bring significant benefits.

- Be patient and kind to yourself. Learning to calm your mind and body takes time and practice.

Enjoy the process of unwinding tension and cultivating inner peace with every breath!

Day 4: Somatic Practices for Digestion & Metabolism - Nurture Your Inner Fire

Welcome to Day 4 of your Somatic Yoga Weight Loss Challenge! Today, we explore mindful movements specifically designed to support healthy digestion and boost metabolism. Remember, our focus is on gentle exploration and listening to your body's unique needs.

Setting the Stage:

- Find a comfortable space free from distractions, with enough room to move freely. You can use a yoga mat or simply practice on the floor.
- Wear loose, comfortable clothing that allows for unrestricted movement.
- Start with a few minutes of mindful breathing, bringing awareness to your breath and allowing your body to settle.

Gentle Twists:

- **Seated Spinal Twists:** Sit comfortably on the floor with your legs crossed or extended in front of you. Gently twist your upper body to one side, placing your hand on your opposite knee for support. Breathe deeply and hold for a few breaths. Repeat on the other side.

- **Standing Twists:** Stand with your feet hip-width apart. Place your hands on your shoulders and gently twist your upper body to one side, keeping your hips facing forward. Breathe deeply and hold for a few breaths. Repeat on the other side.

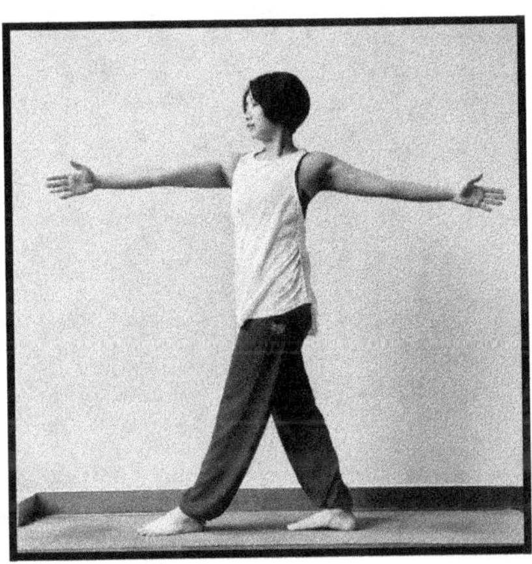

Abdominal Activation:

- **Cat-Cow:** Start on your hands and knees with your back flat and your core engaged. As you inhale, arch your back like a cat, lifting your head and tailbone. As you exhale, round your back, tucking your chin to your chest, and engage your abdominal muscles. Repeat several times, focusing on smooth transitions between poses.

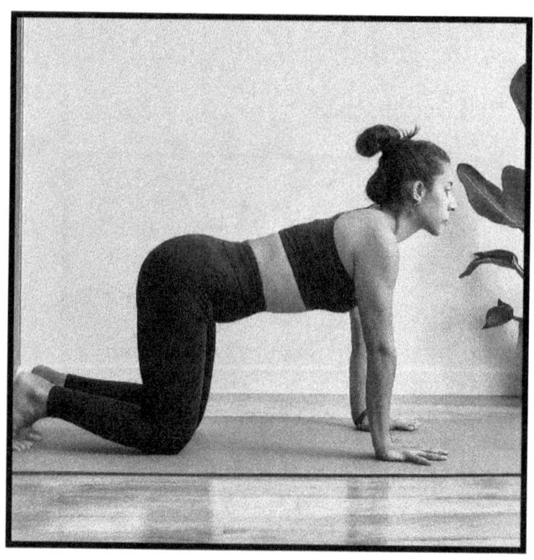

- **Bird-Dog:** Start on your hands and knees with your back flat and your core engaged. Extend one arm forward and the opposite leg back, keeping your spine long and neutral. Hold for a few breaths and then repeat on the other side.

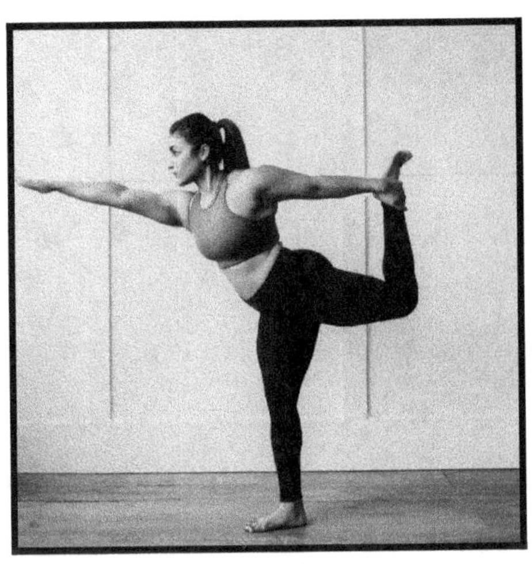

Pelvic Mobility:

- **Pelvic Tilts:** Lie on your back with your knees bent and feet flat on the floor. Gently tilt your pelvis upwards, engaging your lower abdominal muscles. Hold for a few breaths and then release. Repeat a few times.

- **Knee Hugs:** Lie on your back and bring one knee towards your chest, hugging it with both arms. Hold for a few breaths and then gently release. Repeat with the other leg.

Journaling:

- Reflect on your experience today. Did any of the poses feel particularly stimulating or energizing? Did you notice any shifts in your energy levels or digestion?
- Write down a personal intention for incorporating mindful movement into your daily life after meals. Could you do a few seated twists after lunch, take a short walk after dinner, or practice cat-cow on your bed before sleep?

Remember:

- Consistency is key. Even small movements practiced regularly can have a positive impact on your digestion and metabolism.

- Listen to your body and modify any poses as needed. If you experience any pain or discomfort, stop the movement and gently return to a neutral position.
- Enjoy the process and celebrate your progress! By nurturing your inner fire through mindful movement, you're supporting your body's natural ability to function optimally.

Embrace the journey and enjoy the positive effects of Somatic Yoga on your digestion and overall well-being!

Day 5: Rest & Reflection - Integrating New Awareness and Practices

Welcome to Day 5 of your Somatic Yoga Weight Loss Challenge! Today, we take a step back from active movement and devote ourselves to **rest and reflection**. This is a crucial part of the journey, allowing your body and mind to integrate the new experiences and insights gained over the past four days.

Setting the Stage:

- Find a quiet and comfortable space where you won't be disturbed. You can use a yoga mat, blanket, or even your bed.
- Create an ambiance that supports relaxation, such as dimming the lights, playing calming music, or diffusing essential oils.
- Allow yourself to rest in a supported position, lying down on your back or

your side, or sitting comfortably with your spine tall.

- Close your eyes or soften your gaze downwards and take a few deep, mindful breaths.

Reflection:

- Take a mental journey through the past four days of practices. Recall the different body sensations, emotions, and thoughts you experienced.
- Ask yourself questions like:
    - What movements did you find most enjoyable or challenging?
    - Did you discover any areas of tension or limitation in your body?
    - Did you notice any shifts in your energy levels, mood, or digestion?
    - What insights did you gain about your body and its unique needs?

- Journaling can be a powerful tool for reflection. Write down your thoughts, feelings, and observations.

Integration:

- Now, take some time to consider how you can integrate these new learnings into your daily life. Remember, small, sustainable changes are more effective than drastic attempts at overhaul.
- Ask yourself:
    - Which practices resonated most with you?
    - How can you incorporate them into your daily routine, even if it's just for a few minutes each day?
    - Can you use mindful breathwork throughout the day to manage stress?
    - Can you include gentle movements during your workday

to improve your posture and energy levels?

- o Can you apply the principles of awareness and listening to your body to your food choices and eating habits?

Self-Care:

- Remember, rest and self-care are essential aspects of your journey. Schedule time for activities that bring you peace and rejuvenation, like spending time in nature, taking a warm bath, reading a good book, or connecting with loved ones.
- Be kind and compassionate to yourself as you move forward. Progress takes time and consistency, so celebrate your efforts and enjoy the process of creating a healthier, more mindful you.

Looking Ahead:

- Tomorrow, we embark on Week 2 of your Somatic Yoga adventure! Be prepared to explore deeper into building your Somatic Flow with guided sequences and mindful transitions.
- Remember, consistency is key. Commit to showing up for yourself each day, even if it's just for a few minutes of mindful movement or quiet reflection.

Enjoy your well-deserved rest and reflection today! This pause is vital for solidifying your progress and paving the way for a transformative journey ahead.

Day 6: Flowing Sequences & Mindful Transitions - Building Your Somatic Flow

Welcome to Day 6 of your Somatic Yoga Weight Loss Challenge! Today we dive into the heart of **Somatic Flow**, connecting gentle movements into seamless sequences that integrate breath, body, and mind. Remember, prioritize mindful exploration and listen to your body's unique needs.

Setting the Stage:

- **Prepare your space:** Find a quiet, comfortable area with enough room to move freely. You can use a yoga mat or practice barefoot on a soft surface.
- **Warm-up:** Begin with gentle neck rolls, shoulder shrugs, and arm circles to activate your joints and warm up your muscles. Follow with a few rounds of Cat-Cow and pelvic tilts to mobilize your spine and pelvis.

Building Your Somatic Flow:

- **Sun Salutation Flow (Modified):** Adapt the classic Sun Salutation sequence to your comfort level. Here's a basic breakdown:
    - **Mountain Pose:** Stand tall with your feet hip-width apart, arms at your sides.

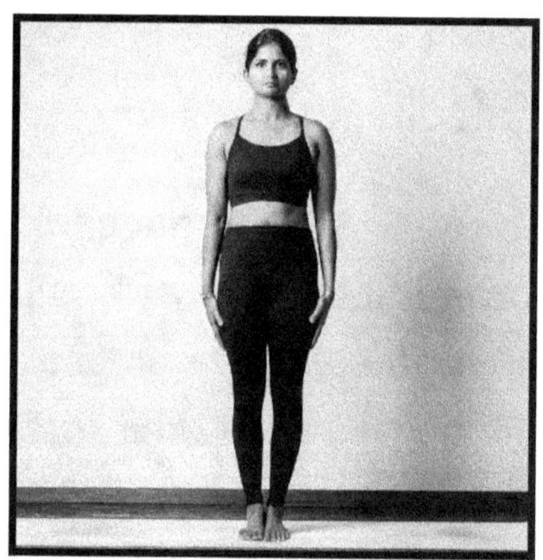

- **Forward Fold:** Hinge at your hips, folding forward with a long spine and reaching towards your shins or floor.

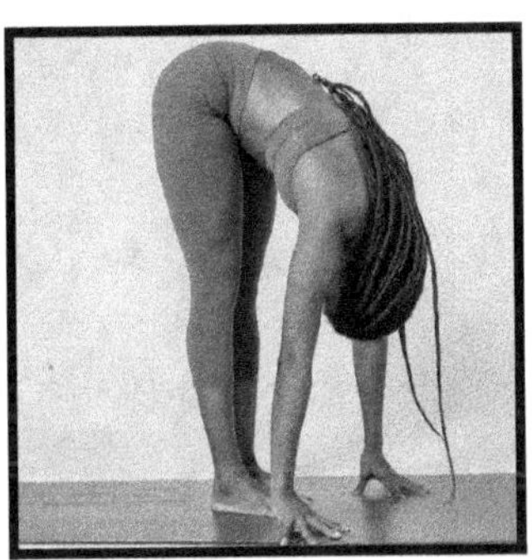

- **Downward-Facing Dog:** Lower your hands shoulder-width apart, push your hips back, and straighten your legs as much as possible, forming an inverted V.

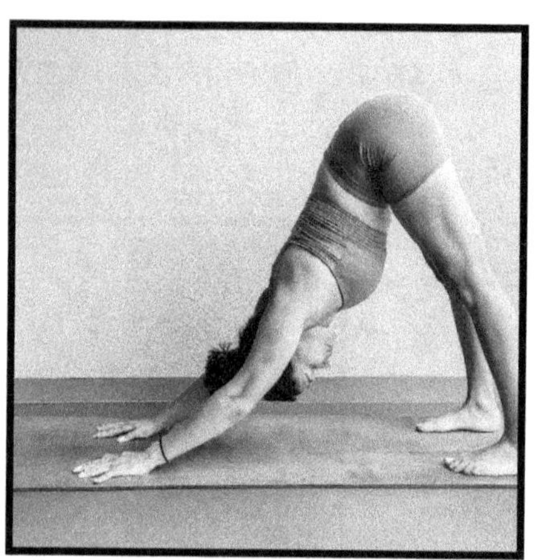

- **Plank:** Lower your body down to a plank position, keeping your core engaged and back flat.

○ **Upward-Facing Dog:** Press your hands and feet into the mat, lift your chest and hips, and arch your back slightly.

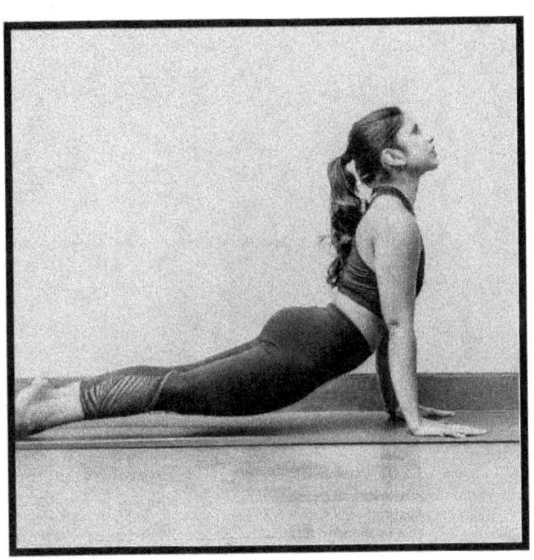

○ **High Lunge:** Step one leg back and lower your hips towards the ground, keeping your front knee bent at a 90-degree angle.

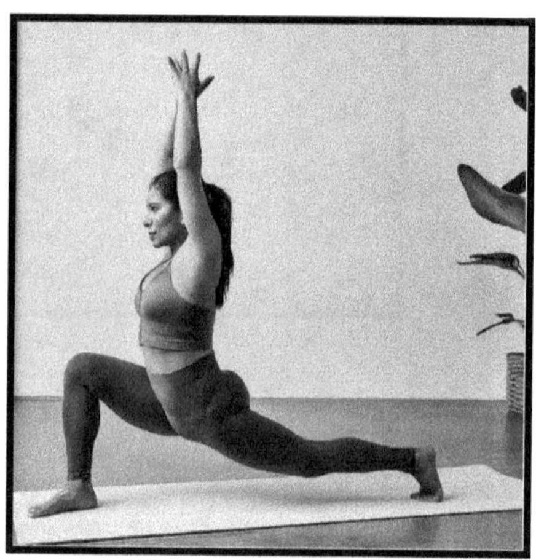

○ **Repeat:** Reverse the sequence, returning to Mountain Pose before transitioning into the next round.

- **Focus on Breath:** Inhale to initiate each movement and exhale as you deepen into the poses. Connect your breath to your movement, creating a smooth and rhythmic flow.
- **Listen to Your Body:** Modify poses as needed. Don't force yourself into anything that feels painful or uncomfortable. Adapt the flow to your own unique limitations and needs.
- **End with Mindfulness:** After completing your flow, lie down in Child's Pose or sit comfortably in Seated Spinal Twists. Allow your body to rest and integrate the experience.

Journaling:

- Reflect on your practice today. What aspects of the flow did you enjoy the most? How did the breath-connected movement feel? Did you encounter any challenges or areas for improvement?

- Write down your observations and insights. This helps you track your progress and solidifies your learning.

Remember:

- Somatic Yoga is a personal journey. Embrace the exploration and celebrate your efforts, regardless of your level of flexibility or experience.
- Consistency is key. Even a short, mindful flow practiced regularly can be more beneficial than occasional intense sessions.
- Enjoy the process of connecting with your body through mindful movement and building your personal Somatic Flow!

Bonus Tip: Incorporate mindful transitions between poses. Observe the space between each movement, feeling the shift in your body and breath. This adds to the meditative quality of your practice.

Have a wonderful Day 6 of your Somatic Yoga journey!

Day 7: Strengthening & Balancing Poses - Engaging Core and Major Muscle Groups

Welcome to Day 7 of your Somatic Yoga Weight Loss Challenge! Today we delve into **strengthening and balancing poses**, gently engaging your major muscle groups while maintaining mindful awareness. Remember, prioritize safe practice and adapt positions as needed.

Setting the Stage:

- **Prepare your space:** Find a comfortable area with enough room to move freely. You can use a yoga mat or practice barefoot on a soft surface.
- **Warm-up:** Repeat the same warm-up routine from Day 6 to activate your joints and warm up your muscles.

Exploring Strengthening Poses:

- **Warrior I & II:** Stand tall with your feet hip-width apart. In Warrior I, step one leg back and bend your front knee, keeping your hips square. In Warrior II, turn your front leg outwards and your back leg inwards, creating a T-shape with your body. Engage your core, lengthen your spine, and hold for a few breaths. Repeat on the other side.

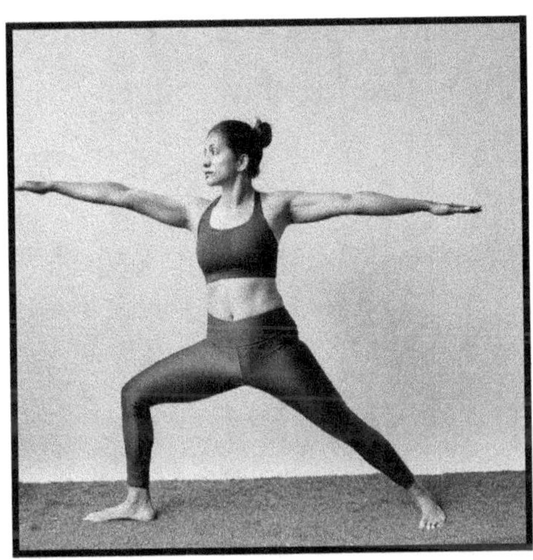

- **Squats:** Stand with your feet hip-width apart and lower your body downwards as if sitting in a chair, keeping your back straight and heels flat on the floor.

Engage your core and glutes to rise back up. You can use a chair for support if needed.

- **Plank Variations:** Start in Downward-Facing Dog and lower your body down to a plank position, keeping your core engaged and back flat. Try different modifications like high plank on your hands, low plank on your forearms, or side planks for an additional core challenge.

Exploring Balancing Poses:

- **Tree Pose:** Stand tall on one leg, bending your other knee and placing your foot on your inner thigh or calf (avoiding the knee joint). Keep your hips level and gaze focused on a point in front of you. Hold for a few breaths and repeat on the other side. You can use a wall or chair for support if needed.

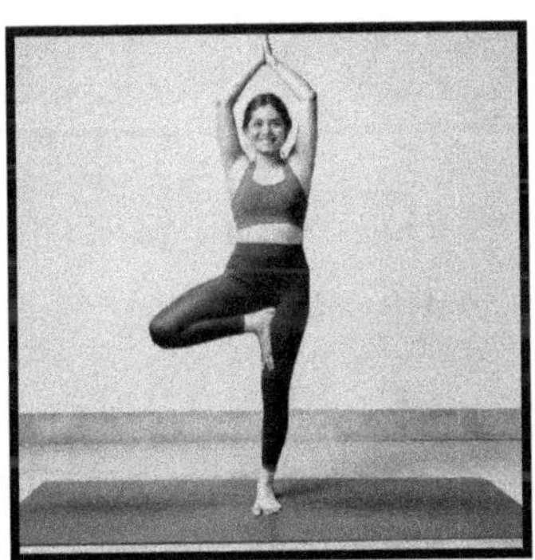

- **Eagle Pose:** Stand tall with your arms outstretched. Bend one knee and wrap it around the other thigh, hooking your foot behind your calf. Wrap your upper arm underneath the opposite arm and gaze focused on a point in front of you. Hold for a few breaths and repeat on the other side.

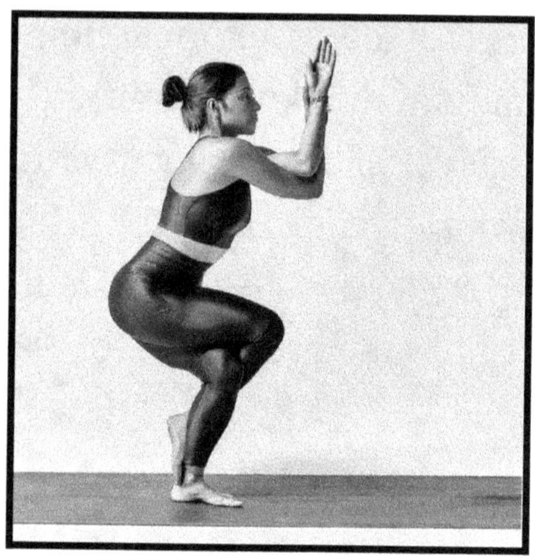

- **Warrior III:** Stand tall on one leg and extend your other leg and arms back, creating a long line from your fingertips to your back heel. Engage your core and gaze focused on a point in front of you. Hold for a few breaths and repeat on the other side.

Cool-down:

- End your practice with Child's Pose or Seated Spinal Twists to allow your body to gently release and integrate the work done.

Journaling:

- Reflect on your experience today. Which poses challenged you the most? Did you discover any areas of weakness or tightness? Were you able to maintain your balance comfortably?
- Write down your observations and insights. This helps you track your progress and identify areas for further focus.

Remember:

- Listen to your body and modify poses as needed. Don't push yourself into

anything that feels painful or
uncomfortable.

- Focus on proper alignment and mindful engagement of your muscles.
- Celebrate your efforts, even if you can't hold poses perfectly. Consistency is key!
- Enjoy the process of strengthening your body and improving your balance with mindful movement.

Bonus Tip: Incorporate mindful transitions between strengthening and balancing poses. Observe the shift in your body and energy as you move from one pose to another. This adds to the meditative quality of your practice.

Have a wonderful and empowering Day 7!

Day 8: Yoga for Stress Management & Emotional Wellbeing - Finding Calm Within

Welcome to Day 8 of your Somatic Yoga Weight Loss Challenge! Today we focus on incorporating **calming Yoga practices** to manage stress and cultivate emotional wellbeing. Remember, prioritize deep relaxation and connecting with your inner peace.

Setting the Stage:

- **Create a calming ambiance:** Dim the lights, light candles or incense, diffuse essential oils, or put on calming music. Choose a quiet, comfortable space where you won't be disturbed.
- **Prepare your body:** Wear loose, comfortable clothing and find a supportive position, like lying down on your back or sitting comfortably with your spine tall.

- **Begin with mindful breathing:** Close your eyes or soften your gaze downwards. Take a few deep, slow breaths, focusing on the rise and fall of your chest and abdomen. Notice any tension or resistance in your body and allow it to soften with each exhale.

Restorative Poses:

- **Supported Child's Pose:** Fold forward with your head resting on a bolster or pillow, arms alongside your body or reaching forward. Let your forehead sink into the support and allow your body to completely relax. Stay for 5-10 minutes.
- **Legs-Up-the-Wall Pose:** Prop your legs up against a wall, creating a 90-degree angle with your torso. Close your eyes, relax your arms at your sides, and breathe deeply for 5-10 minutes.

- **Supported Savasana:** Lie down on your back with a bolster or pillows placed under your knees and head for support. Allow your arms to rest at your sides and your body to melt into the support. Stay for 10-15 minutes.

Guided Meditation (Yoga Nidra):

Find a guided Yoga Nidra meditation online or use a meditation app. Nidra is a deeply relaxing guided practice that leads you through visualization and body awareness techniques to promote inner peace and stress reduction. Aim for 15-20 minutes of guided meditation.

Journaling:

- Reflect on your experience today. How did the restorative poses affect your body and mind? Did you observe any shifts in your emotions or stress levels? How did the meditation feel?

- Write down your thoughts, feelings, and insights. This helps you process your experience and identify areas for continued growth.

Remember:

- Finding inner peace is a journey, not a destination. Be patient with yourself and celebrate your efforts, even if you don't feel completely calm at first.
- Consistency is key. Even a few minutes of calming Yoga practice each day can have a significant impact on your stress levels and emotional wellbeing.
- Be kind and compassionate to yourself. Remember, stress management is a continuous process, and setbacks are normal.
- Enjoy the process of cultivating inner peace and finding your path to emotional wellbeing through mindful movement and meditation.

Bonus Tip: Throughout the day, incorporate mindful breathing exercises whenever you feel stressed or overwhelmed. Take a few deep breaths, focusing on your inhale and exhale, to calm your mind and body.

Have a peaceful and mindful Day 8!

Day 9: Exploring Poses for Flexibility & Range of Motion - Expanding Your Boundaries (Respectfully)

Welcome to Day 9 of your Somatic Yoga Weight Loss Challenge! Today, we dive into **exploring poses that gently improve your flexibility and range of motion**, respecting your body's unique limitations and honoring its signals. Remember, prioritize mindful exploration and safety over forcing yourself into uncomfortable positions.

Setting the Stage:

- **Prepare your space:** Find a comfortable area with enough room to move freely. You can use a yoga mat or practice barefoot on a soft surface.
- **Warm-up:** Repeat the same warm-up routine from Day 6 to activate your joints and warm up your muscles.

Exploring Flexibility Poses:

- **Forward Bends:**
  - **Seated Forward Bend:** Sit on the floor with your legs extended and reach forward towards your shins or toes. Keep your spine long and hinge at your hips, not your lower back. Hold for a few breaths.
  - **Standing Forward Bend:** Stand tall with your feet hip-width apart and hinge forward, folding over your legs. Allow your head to hang heavy and soften your knees if needed. Hold for a few breaths.
  - **Pyramid Pose:** Stand with your feet wider than hip-width apart and reach one hand down towards your shin or ankle, keeping the other leg straight. Keep your spine long and gaze towards your front hand. Hold for

a few breaths and repeat on the other side.

- **Hip Openers:**
  - **Half Pigeon Pose:** Start in Downward-Facing Dog and bring one knee forward between your hands. Lower your hips towards the floor and lengthen your back leg. Stay for a few breaths and repeat on the other side.
  - **Figure-Four Pose:** Lie on your back and cross one ankle over the opposite thigh, hooking your foot behind your calf. Gently pull your thigh towards your chest and hold for a few breaths. Repeat on the other side.
  - **Lizard Pose:** Start in Downward-Facing Dog and step one leg forward between your hands. Lower your hips towards the floor and keep your back leg

straight. Stay for a few breaths and repeat on the other side.

Cool-down:

- End your practice with Child's Pose or Seated Spinal Twists to allow your body to gently release and integrate the work done.

Journaling:

- Reflect on your experience today. Which poses challenged your flexibility the most? Did you discover any areas of tightness or limitation? Were you able to maintain gentle length without forcing anything?
- Write down your observations and insights. This helps you track your progress and identify areas for further focus.

Remember:

- **Listen to your body:** It's your guide. Don't push yourself beyond your comfortable range of motion. If you feel pain, stop the pose and gently come out of it.
- **Focus on mindfulness:** Pay attention to your breath and body sensations throughout each pose. Observe where you hold tension and try to release it with each exhale.
- **Celebrate small improvements:** Flexibility takes time and consistent practice. Don't get discouraged if you can't reach your toes today. Be proud of the progress you make, even if it's small.
- **Enjoy the journey:** Exploring flexibility with mindfulness is a rewarding experience. Connect with your body, embrace its unique needs, and enjoy the feeling of increased ease and movement.

Bonus Tip: Incorporate mindful stretches throughout your day. Reach for your toes while sitting at your desk, roll your shoulders while waiting in line, or gently twist your torso while watching TV. These small movements can help improve your flexibility over time.

Have a mindful and empowering Day 9!

Day 10: Rest & Recharge - Deepening Your Connection to Self

Welcome to Day 10 of your Somatic Yoga Weight Loss Challenge! Today, we take a step back from active movement and dedicate time for **rest and reflection**, deepening your connection to your body and the journey you're on. Remember, rest is as important as movement in nurturing overall well-being.

Setting the Stage:

- Create a **peaceful and supportive environment**. Dim the lights, light candles or incense, play calming music, or simply find a quiet, comfortable space where you won't be disturbed.
- **Allow yourself to rest:** Choose a restful position that works for you, whether it's lying down in Savasana, sitting comfortably in meditation, or simply reclining on a sofa or in a hammock.

- **Practice mindful breathing:** Close your eyes or soften your gaze downwards. Take a few deep, slow breaths, focusing on the rise and fall of your chest and abdomen. Observe any tension or resistance in your body and allow it to soften with each exhale.

Reflection and Journaling:

- Take a mental journey through the past nine days of practices. Recall the different body sensations, emotions, and thoughts you experienced.
- Ask yourself questions like:
    - What aspects of the practices did you enjoy the most?
    - Did you discover any areas of tension or limitation in your body?
    - Did you notice any shifts in your energy levels, mood, or digestion?

- What insights did you gain about your body and its unique needs?
    - How has your overall outlook on your weight loss journey shifted?
- Journaling can be a powerful tool for reflection. Write down your thoughts, feelings, and observations. This helps you integrate your experiences and solidify your learnings.

Setting Intentions:

- Now, take some time to consider how you can **integrate these new learnings into your life beyond the challenge**. Remember, small, sustainable changes are more effective than drastic attempts at overhaul.
- Ask yourself:
    - Which practices resonated most with you?
    - How can you incorporate mindful movement into your daily

routine, even if it's just for a few
minutes each day?

- o Can you use breathwork
  throughout the day to manage
  stress?
- o Can you apply the principles of
  awareness and listening to your
  body to your food choices and
  eating habits?
- o How can you prioritize self-care
  and rest in your daily life?

- Create realistic and personalized
  intentions for your well-being moving
  forward. Remember, consistency is
  key, even if it's just small steps or
  moments of mindful awareness.

Embrace the Journey:

- This challenge is not about reaching a
  specific destination, but rather about
  embarking on a continuous journey of
  self-discovery and mindful movement.

Celebrate your progress, big or small, and be patient with yourself.

- Remember, self-compassion is key. Be kind to yourself as you navigate challenges and setbacks.
- Take the learnings and tools you gained from this challenge and integrate them into your life in a way that feels authentic and sustainable.

Enjoy your well-deserved rest and reflection today! This pause is vital for solidifying your progress and paving the way for a transformative journey ahead.

Remember, this is just the beginning of your Somatic Yoga journey. Continue to explore, listen to your body, and enjoy the process of connecting with your inner wisdom and achieving your well-being goals.

Chapter 3

Week 3: Deepening Your Practice

While Day 11 of the Somatic Yoga Weight Loss Challenge is listed as focusing on targeted poses for abdominal strengthening, it's important to remember that **spot reduction (reducing fat in specific areas) is not possible**. Overall healthy eating and consistent exercise contribute to fat loss throughout the body, including the abdomen. However, Somatic Yoga practices can strengthen and tone your core muscles, improving posture, stability, and overall well-being.

Here are some **Somatic Yoga principles** to remember before exploring poses:

- **Focus on mindful movement:** Pay attention to your breath, body sensations, and alignment throughout each pose.
- **Listen to your body:** Don't force yourself into anything uncomfortable or painful. Modify poses as needed.
- **Engage your core:** Activate your core muscles during all poses, not just those specifically targeting the abdomen.
- **Breathe deeply:** Coordinate your breath with your movement for deeper engagement and relaxation.

Now, let's explore some **Somatic Yoga poses** that can help strengthen your core:

Warm-up:

- **Cat-Cow:** Move your spine into a gentle arch (cow) and round (cat) while coordinating your breath.

- **Pelvic tilts:** Tilt your pelvis forward and backward, feeling the engagement in your core and lower back.
- **Arm circles:** Forward and backward circles with your arms to warm up your shoulders and torso.

Core-Engaging Poses:

- **Plank:** Start on your forearms and knees, then lift your knees off the ground to form a straight line from head to heels. Engage your core to keep your back flat and hips stable. Modify on your knees if needed.
- **Side plank:** Start on your forearm and side of your foot, lifting your hips off the ground. Stack your shoulders, hips, and ankles in a straight line. Hold on each side.
- **Boat pose:** Sit on your tailbone with legs extended and lifted off the ground, back leaning slightly back. Reach your

arms forward and engage your core for balance.

- **Bird-dog:** Start on all fours, extend one arm forward and the opposite leg back, keeping your back flat and core engaged. Repeat on the other side.

Cool-down:

- **Child's pose:** Rest your forehead on the mat with your hips back and arms alongside your body. Breathe deeply and release any tension.
- **Seated spinal twists:** Gently twist your upper body to each side, keeping your hips grounded. Breathe deeply into each twist.

Remember:

- Consistency is key. Even a few minutes of mindful core engagement each day can benefit your overall well-being.

- Combine core-strengthening exercises with a balanced diet and other forms of exercise for optimal results.
- Celebrate your progress and enjoy the journey of connecting with your body through mindful movement.

I hope this information helps you explore core-strengthening practices in a safe and mindful way!

While Day 11 of the Somatic Yoga Weight Loss Challenge is listed as focusing on targeted poses for abdominal strengthening, it's important to remember that **spot reduction (reducing fat in specific areas) is not possible**. Overall healthy eating and consistent exercise contribute to fat loss throughout the body, including the abdomen. However, Somatic Yoga practices can strengthen and tone your core muscles, improving posture, stability, and overall well-being.

Here are some **Somatic Yoga principles** to remember before exploring poses:

- **Focus on mindful movement:** Pay attention to your breath, body sensations, and alignment throughout each pose.
- **Listen to your body:** Don't force yourself into anything uncomfortable or painful. Modify poses as needed.
- **Engage your core:** Activate your core muscles during all poses, not just those specifically targeting the abdomen.
- **Breathe deeply:** Coordinate your breath with your movement for deeper engagement and relaxation.

Now, let's explore some **Somatic Yoga poses** that can help strengthen your core:

Warm-up:

- **Cat-Cow:** Move your spine into a gentle arch (cow) and round (cat) while coordinating your breath.
- **Pelvic tilts:** Tilt your pelvis forward and backward, feeling the engagement in your core and lower back.
- **Arm circles:** Forward and backward circles with your arms to warm up your shoulders and torso.

Core-Engaging Poses:

- **Plank:** Start on your forearms and knees, then lift your knees off the ground to form a straight line from head to heels. Engage your core to keep your back flat and hips stable. Modify on your knees if needed.
- **Side plank:** Start on your forearm and side of your foot, lifting your hips off the ground. Stack your shoulders, hips, and ankles in a straight line. Hold on each side.

- **Boat pose:** Sit on your tailbone with legs extended and lifted off the ground, back leaning slightly back. Reach your arms forward and engage your core for balance.
- **Bird-dog:** Start on all fours, extend one arm forward and the opposite leg back, keeping your back flat and core engaged. Repeat on the other side.

Cool-down:

- **Child's pose:** Rest your forehead on the mat with your hips back and arms alongside your body. Breathe deeply and release any tension.
- **Seated spinal twists:** Gently twist your upper body to each side, keeping your hips grounded. Breathe deeply into each twist.

Remember:

- Consistency is key. Even a few minutes of mindful core engagement each day can benefit your overall well-being.
- Combine core-strengthening exercises with a balanced diet and other forms of exercise for optimal results.
- Celebrate your progress and enjoy the journey of connecting with your body through mindful movement.

I hope this information helps you explore core-strengthening practices in a safe and mindful way!

Day 12: Yoga for Healthy Eating Habits & Mindful Food Choices - Cultivating Inner Wisdom on Your Plate

Welcome to Day 12 of your Somatic Yoga Weight Loss Challenge! Today, we delve into the **connection between Yoga and mindful eating**, exploring practices that cultivate awareness and support healthy food choices. Remember, the focus is on building a positive and intuitive relationship with food.

Setting the Stage:

- Create a **calm and distraction-free environment** for your practice. Dim the lights, light candles, or play calming music. Sit comfortably on a chair or cushion with your back straight.
- **Begin with mindful breathing:** Close your eyes or soften your gaze downwards. Take a few deep, slow breaths, focusing on the rise and fall of

your chest and abdomen. Observe any tension or resistance in your body and allow it to soften with each exhale.

Explore Mindful Eating Practices:

- **Body Scan:** Gently bring your awareness to different parts of your body, starting with your toes and moving upwards. Notice any sensations of hunger, fullness, or cravings without judgment.
- **Visualization:** Imagine yourself making healthy food choices. Visualize the colors, textures, and smells of nourishing foods that make you feel good.
- **Affirmations:** Repeat positive affirmations about yourself and your relationship with food, like "I choose to nourish my body with healthy foods" or "I trust my body's signals."

- **Gratitude Exercise:** Before eating, take a moment to appreciate the food you have. Consider the farmers, chefs, and everyone involved in bringing it to your table.

Connect with Your Inner Wisdom:

- **Ask yourself questions:** Before reaching for food, ask yourself if you're truly hungry or seeking emotional comfort. Is this the best choice for your body and well-being?
- **Pay attention to internal cues:** Notice your body's signals of hunger, fullness, and satisfaction. Stop eating when you're comfortably full, not stuffed.
- **Challenge emotional eating:** Identify triggers for emotional eating and explore mindful breathing techniques or other practices to manage stress and emotions without turning to food for comfort.

Yoga Poses for Grounding and Awareness:

- **Mountain Pose:** Stand tall with your feet hip-width apart, arms at your sides. Feel rooted and grounded to the earth.
- **Tree Pose:** Stand on one leg, raising the other foot to rest on your inner thigh or calf. Hold for a few breaths and repeat on the other side. Focus on balance and stability.
- **Child's Pose:** Kneel on the floor with your toes together and sit back on your heels. Rest your forehead on the mat and allow your arms to relax alongside your body. Feel supported and connected to the earth.

Journaling:

- Reflect on your experience today. How did the mindfulness practices impact your awareness of your body and food choices? Did you observe any new insights about your eating habits?

- Write down your thoughts, feelings, and observations. This helps you track your progress and identify areas for continued awareness.

Remember:

- Building a healthy relationship with food takes time and practice. Be patient with yourself and celebrate your efforts, even small shifts in awareness.
- Yoga is a tool to support your journey, not a quick fix. Combine mindful eating practices with a balanced diet and other self-care activities for optimal well-being.
- Enjoy the process of connecting with your body's wisdom and making food choices that nourish your mind, body, and soul.

Bonus Tip: Practice mindful eating throughout the day. Pay attention to how you feel before, during, and after eating. This awareness can help you make choices that align with your well-being goals.

Have a mindful and empowering Day 12!

Day 13: Restorative Poses for Stress Release & Recovery

Welcome to Day 13 of your Somatic Yoga Weight Loss Challenge! Today, we take a well-deserved pause for **rest and recovery** with soothing **restorative Yoga poses**. Remember, rest is just as important as movement in your overall well-being journey.

Setting the Stage:

- Create a **calming and supportive environment**. Dim the lights, light candles or incense, play relaxing music, or simply find a quiet, comfortable space where you won't be disturbed.
- **Gather props:** Bolsters, pillows, blankets, and straps can enhance your comfort and deepen your relaxation in the poses.
- **Prepare your body:** Wear loose, comfortable clothing and choose a

restful position, like lying down on your back or sitting comfortably with your spine tall.

- **Begin with mindful breathing:** Close your eyes or soften your gaze downwards. Take a few deep, slow breaths, focusing on the rise and fall of your chest and abdomen. Observe any tension or resistance in your body and allow it to soften with each exhale.

Restorative Poses:

- **Supported Child's Pose:** Fold forward with your head resting on a bolster or pillow, arms alongside your body or reaching forward. Let your forehead sink into the support and allow your body to completely relax. Stay for 5-10 minutes.
- **Legs-Up-the-Wall Pose:** Prop your legs up against a wall, creating a 90-degree angle with your torso. Close

your eyes, relax your arms at your sides, and breathe deeply for 5-10 minutes.

- **Supported Savasana:** Lie down on your back with bolsters or pillows placed under your knees and head for support. Allow your arms to rest at your sides and your body to melt into the support. Stay for 10-15 minutes.
- **Supine Spinal Twist (optional):** Lie on your back with your knees bent and feet flat on the floor. Gently lower one knee to the opposite side of your body, resting it near your armpit. Turn your head in the opposite direction and allow your gaze to soften. Hold for a few breaths and repeat on the other side.

Deepen Your Relaxation:

- **Use guided meditation:** Find a guided meditation online or use a meditation app specifically for relaxation. 10-15 minutes of guided meditation can further deepen your rest and release stress.

- **Focus on your breath:** Throughout the poses, maintain slow, deep breaths. Observe the natural rhythm of your breath and allow it to carry away any tension.
- **Practice self-compassion:** Be kind to yourself and allow your body to receive the rest it needs.

After Your Practice:

- Take a few moments to come out of the poses slowly and mindfully.
- Journal about your experience. Did you notice any shifts in your body or mind? How did you feel before and after the practice?
- Reflect on your progress so far in the challenge. What have you learned?

What challenges did you overcome? Celebrate your achievements!

Remember:

- Rest is essential for physical and mental well-being. Make it a priority in your overall health journey.
- Restorative Yoga can be a powerful tool for stress relief and recovery. Integrate it into your routine whenever needed.
- Be patient and kind to yourself. Finding balance and inner peace takes time and consistent effort.

Enjoy your restorative rest and remember, **self-care is not selfish, it's essential!**

Day 14: Building Stamina & Endurance with Somatic Flow

Welcome to Day 14 of your Somatic Yoga Weight Loss Challenge! Today, we focus on **building stamina and endurance** while maintaining mindful movement with **Somatic Flow**. Remember, prioritize smooth transitions and listen to your body's needs throughout the practice.

Setting the Stage:

- Find a comfortable space with enough room to move freely. You can use a yoga mat or practice barefoot on a soft surface.
- Warm up your body with gentle neck rolls, shoulder shrugs, arm circles, and a few rounds of Cat-Cow and pelvic tilts.
- Connect to your breath. Take a few deep, mindful breaths to calm your mind and center yourself.

Building Stamina with Flow:

- **Start with familiar sequences:** Begin with modified Sun Salutations or other flows you practiced earlier in the challenge. Focus on smooth transitions and connecting each breath to your movement.

- **Gradually increase repetitions:** Once you feel comfortable with a sequence, try adding one or two more repetitions for each pose. Observe how your body feels and adjust as needed.

- **Explore dynamic variations:** Experiment with adding dynamic movements within poses, like jumping jacks in Downward-Facing Dog or lunges in Warrior II. Remember to maintain proper form and prioritize mindful transitions.

- **Incorporate longer holds:** Hold poses for a few breaths longer than usual to challenge your stamina and build strength. Listen to your body and don't push yourself to the point of discomfort.

Maintaining Mindful Awareness:

- **Focus on your breath:** Pay attention to your inhale and exhale throughout the flow. Use your breath to guide your movement and deepen your focus.
- **Listen to your body:** Don't push yourself beyond your limits. If you feel pain or discomfort, modify the pose or take a break. Remember, progress is gradual, not forced.
- **Celebrate small victories:** Be proud of yourself for showing up and practicing, even if you can't hold poses for long or complete the entire flow without modifications. Every effort counts!

Cool-down and Reflection:

- After your flow, end with Child's Pose or Seated Spinal Twists to allow your body to gently release and integrate the work done.
- Take a few moments to reflect on your experience. How did your body feel during the flow? Did you notice any improvements in your stamina or endurance? What challenges did you encounter?
- Journal about your observations and insights. This helps you track your progress and identify areas for further focus.

Remember:

- Building stamina takes time and consistent practice. Be patient with yourself and celebrate your progress, no matter how small.

- Listen to your body and prioritize mindful movement over forcing yourself into challenging positions.
- Combine your Somatic Flow practice with other activities like brisk walking, swimming, or cycling for a well-rounded approach to improving your cardiovascular health and endurance.
- Most importantly, enjoy the process of moving your body with awareness and building your inner strength!

Bonus Tip: Incorporate mindful movement throughout your day. Take the stairs instead of the elevator, do some stretches while waiting in line, or park further away and walk to your destination. These small movements contribute to your overall stamina and well-being.

Have a mindful and empowering Day 14!

Welcome to Day 15 of your Somatic Yoga Weight Loss Challenge! Today marks a significant milestone in your journey – 15 days filled with mindful movement, exploration, and self-discovery.

It's time to **pause, reflect, and celebrate** all that you've accomplished!

Celebrate Your Success:

- **Reflect on your starting point:** How did you feel when you began this challenge? What were your goals and intentions?
- **Acknowledge your progress:** Take a moment to appreciate the efforts you've put in, big or small. Did you notice any improvements in your flexibility, strength, or overall well-being? Did you discover new insights about your body and mind?
- **Feel proud of yourself:** Acknowledge your commitment and dedication to

prioritizing your health and well-being through mindful movement.

Set New Goals:

- **Consider your journey so far:** What practices resonated most with you? What aspects did you find challenging? How do you want to continue incorporating Somatic Yoga into your life beyond the challenge?
- **Set realistic and achievable goals:** Think about specific practices you want to continue or integrate into your routine. Consider focusing on specific areas you want to work on, like improving your balance or increasing your flexibility in certain poses.
- **Write down your goals:** This helps solidify your intentions and make them more concrete. Remember, small, sustainable changes are more effective than drastic attempts at overhaul.

Embrace the Journey:

- **Remember, this is a continuous journey, not a destination.** Celebrate your progress along the way, and be patient with yourself on days when you face challenges or setbacks.
- **Stay inspired and motivated:** There are endless resources available to continue your exploration of Somatic Yoga. Explore online classes, workshops, or find a local studio that aligns with your interests.
- **Most importantly, enjoy the process!** Find joy in moving your body with awareness, connecting with your breath, and nurturing your overall well-being through mindful movement.

Beyond Day 15:

As you step beyond Day 15, remember that **Somatic Yoga is a philosophy and practice that extends beyond this specific challenge.**

Continue to explore, listen to your body, and enjoy the journey of connecting with your inner wisdom and achieving your well-being goals.

Here are some additional thoughts to keep in mind:

- **Combine Somatic Yoga with other healthy habits:** Maintain a balanced diet, get enough sleep, and manage stress effectively for optimal well-being.
- **Listen to your body and modify as needed:** Every body is unique and has different needs. Don't push yourself beyond your limits and always prioritize safety and mindful movement.
- **Be kind and compassionate to yourself:** This is a journey of exploration and self-discovery, not a competition. Celebrate your progress

and be patient with yourself on challenging days.

Congratulations on completing this 15-day challenge! Carry the learnings, insights, and joy of movement forward as you continue on your path to well-being. Remember, every step you take, every mindful breath you connect with, is a step towards a more empowered and healthy you.

Day 15: Rest & Reflect - Celebrating Progress and Setting New Goals

Welcome to Day 15 of your Somatic Yoga Weight Loss Challenge! Today marks a significant milestone in your journey – 15 days filled with mindful movement, exploration, and self-discovery.

It's time to **pause, reflect, and celebrate** all that you've accomplished!

Celebrate Your Success:

- **Reflect on your starting point:** How did you feel when you began this challenge? What were your goals and intentions?
- **Acknowledge your progress:** Take a moment to appreciate the efforts you've put in, big or small. Did you notice any improvements in your flexibility, strength, or overall well-being? Did

you discover new insights about your body and mind?

- **Feel proud of yourself:** Acknowledge your commitment and dedication to prioritizing your health and well-being through mindful movement.

Set New Goals:

- **Consider your journey so far:** What practices resonated most with you? What aspects did you find challenging? How do you want to continue incorporating Somatic Yoga into your life beyond the challenge?
- **Set realistic and achievable goals:** Think about specific practices you want to continue or integrate into your routine. Consider focusing on specific areas you want to work on, like improving your balance or increasing your flexibility in certain poses.

- **Write down your goals:** This helps solidify your intentions and make them more concrete. Remember, small, sustainable changes are more effective than drastic attempts at overhaul.

Embrace the Journey:

- **Remember, this is a continuous journey, not a destination.** Celebrate your progress along the way, and be patient with yourself on days when you face challenges or setbacks.
- **Stay inspired and motivated:** There are endless resources available to continue your exploration of Somatic Yoga. Explore online classes, workshops, or find a local studio that aligns with your interests.
- **Most importantly, enjoy the process!** Find joy in moving your body with awareness, connecting with your

breath, and nurturing your overall well-being through mindful movement.

Beyond Day 15:

As you step beyond Day 15, remember that **Somatic Yoga is a philosophy and practice that extends beyond this specific challenge.** Continue to explore, listen to your body, and enjoy the journey of connecting with your inner wisdom and achieving your well-being goals.

Here are some additional thoughts to keep in mind:

- **Combine Somatic Yoga with other healthy habits:** Maintain a balanced diet, get enough sleep, and manage stress effectively for optimal well-being.
- **Listen to your body and modify as needed:** Every body is unique and has different needs. Don't push yourself

beyond your limits and always prioritize safety and mindful movement.

- **Be kind and compassionate to yourself:** This is a journey of exploration and self-discovery, not a competition. Celebrate your progress and be patient with yourself on challenging days.

Congratulations on completing this 15-day challenge! Carry the learnings, insights, and joy of movement forward as you continue on your path to well-being. Remember, every step you take, every mindful breath you connect with, is a step towards a more empowered and healthy you.

Chapter 4

Week 4: Sustaining Your Transformation

Day 16: Creating a Personalized Somatic Yoga Routine

Sure, creating a personalized Somatic Yoga routine is a great way to continue your practice and reap the benefits of mindful movement. Here are some steps to get you started:

1. **Reflect on your experience.** Think about what you enjoyed most about the 15-day challenge. Did you find certain poses or practices particularly helpful? What areas would you like to focus on moving forward?

2. **Set realistic goals.** Don't try to do too much too soon. Start with a few poses or practices that you can commit to

doing regularly. You can gradually add more as you get stronger and more comfortable.

3. **Consider your time constraints.** How much time do you realistically have to devote to your practice each day? Even 10-15 minutes can make a difference.

4. **Find a space that you enjoy.** Your practice space should be quiet, comfortable, and free from distractions.

5. **Gather the props you need.** You may need a yoga mat, blocks, blankets, or bolsters.

6. **Warm up before you begin.** This will help to prevent injuries.

7. **Listen to your body.** Don't push yourself beyond your limits. If you feel pain, stop the pose and rest.

8. **Be patient and consistent.** It takes time to see results from any exercise program. Stick with it and you will eventually see and feel the benefits.

Here is a sample Somatic Yoga routine that you can modify to fit your needs:

- **Warm-up:** 5-10 minutes of gentle stretches and movements, such as neck rolls, shoulder shrugs, arm circles, and Cat-Cow pose.
- **Sun Salutations:** 3-5 rounds of modified Sun Salutations.
- **Standing poses:** Warrior I, Warrior II, Triangle pose, Tree pose, Half Moon pose (optional).
- **Seated poses:** Seated Forward Fold, Seated Twist, Hero pose.
- **Supine poses:** Child's pose, Bridge pose, Supported Savasana.
- **Cool-down:** 5-10 minutes of gentle stretches and relaxation poses, such as Child's pose and Savasana.

You can also find many online resources for creating personalized Somatic Yoga routines. Here are a few of my favorites:

- **DoYogaWithMe:** [https www doyogawithme com]
- **Yoga Journal:** [https www yogajournal com]
- **Ekhart Yoga:** [https www ekhartyoga com]

I hope this helps!

Day 17: Yoga for Maintaining Motivation & Overcoming Challenges - Fueling Your Inner Spark

Welcome to Day 17! As your Somatic Yoga journey continues, remember, maintaining motivation and navigating challenges are essential parts of any long-term endeavor. Today, we explore practices that cultivate resilience and rekindle your inner spark for mindful movement.

Setting the Stage:

- Create a **calming and supportive environment**. Dim the lights, light candles, or play calming music. Choose a spot free from distractions where you can connect with yourself fully.
- **Begin with grounding poses:** Start with Mountain Pose or Downward-Facing Dog to feel rooted and present. Take a few deep, mindful

breaths, focusing on your inhale and exhale.

- **Set your intention:** Before starting your practice, set an intention for yourself. Perhaps it's "to rediscover joy in movement" or "to overcome resistance with gentle awareness."

Exploring Practices for Motivation:

- **Dynamic Flow:** Engage in a short flow sequence, like Sun Salutations or a creative sequence you enjoy. Feel the energy flowing through your body and connect with your breath.
- **Heart-Opening Poses:** Practice poses like Camel Pose, Bridge Pose, or Warrior II variations that open your chest and heart center. Allow yourself to feel empowered and inspired.
- **Inversions (optional):** If comfortable, explore gentle inversions like Downward-Facing Dog or Supported

Headstand. These poses can shift your perspective and boost energy levels.

- **Gratitude Practice:** During or after your practice, take a moment to express gratitude for your body, its capabilities, and the opportunity to move. Acknowledge your efforts and progress.

Overcoming Challenges:

- **Identify your obstacles:** Reflect on what hinders your motivation. Is it time constraints, self-doubt, lack of inspiration, or something else? Recognizing the challenge is the first step towards overcoming it.
- **Embrace small wins:** Celebrate every step forward, no matter how small. Completing a short practice, trying a new pose, or simply showing up on your mat are all victories worthy of appreciation.

- **Seek support:** Connect with a yoga community online or in person. Share your experiences, draw inspiration from others, and offer support in return.
- **Modify when needed:** Don't be afraid to modify poses or shorten your practice when needed. Prioritize listening to your body and creating a sustainable practice that works for you.
- **Remember your "why":** Recall your initial motivation for starting Somatic Yoga. What were your goals and desires? Reconnecting with your "why" can reignite your passion and commitment.

Remember:

- **Motivation fluctuates:** It's normal to experience ups and downs. Accept that there will be days when movement feels effortless and others when it requires more effort. Be kind to yourself throughout the journey.

- **Focus on progress, not perfection:** Every practice is an opportunity to learn and grow. Don't compare yourself to others or get discouraged by setbacks. Celebrate your unique journey.
- **Enjoy the process:** Find joy in the movement itself, the connection with your breath, and the exploration of your inner world. Let Somatic Yoga be a source of nourishment for your mind, body, and spirit.

Bonus Tip: Incorporate mindful moments throughout your day. Take a few deep breaths when feeling stressed, stretch your body while waiting in line, or simply notice the sensations in your feet as you walk. These small moments of awareness can keep you connected to your practice and cultivate motivation for your next session.

Day 18: Integrating Somatic Practices into Daily Life - Weaving Mindfulness into Your Journey

Welcome to Day 18! As you complete this Somatic Yoga exploration, it's time to **integrate its essence into your daily life**, making mindful movement and awareness a natural part of your routine. Remember, it's not about perfection, but about cultivating sustainable practices that nurture your well-being.

Exploring Integration Points:

- **Mindful Movement Throughout the Day:**
  - Incorporate micro-stretches while waiting in line, sitting at your desk, or watching TV.
  - Take the stairs instead of the elevator, do some gentle shoulder rolls while talking on the phone,

or simply stand tall and grounded for a few minutes.

  - Practice mindful walking, focusing on the sensations in your feet and body with each step.

- **Mindful Breathing:**
  - Throughout the day, take a few conscious breaths whenever you feel stressed, overwhelmed, or need a moment of pause.
  - Use your breath to calm your mind and connect with your physical presence.
  - Explore simple breathing exercises like alternate nostril breathing or box breathing for quick stress relief.

- **Mindful Eating:**
  - Before eating, pause and take a few mindful breaths. Ask

yourself if you're truly hungry or seeking emotional comfort.

   o Eat slowly and savor each bite, paying attention to the taste, texture, and aroma of your food.

   o Stop eating when you're comfortably full, not stuffed.

- **Mindful Body Scans:**

   o Take a few minutes throughout the day to do a mindful body scan, bringing your awareness to different parts of your body and noticing any sensations without judgment.

   o This practice can help you release tension, improve body awareness, and cultivate inner peace.

Building Sustainable Habits:

- **Start small and consistent:** Don't try to overwhelm yourself. Begin with incorporating one or two practices into your daily routine and gradually build from there.

- **Find activities you enjoy:** Explore different mindful movement practices until you find ones you truly connect with and enjoy.
- **Pair practices with existing routines:** Integrate mindful movement into your daily activities. Do some stretches while waiting for your coffee, practice mindful breathing during your commute, or take a mindful walk during your lunch break.
- **Track your progress:** Keep a journal or use a habit tracker app to monitor your progress and celebrate your achievements. This can help maintain motivation and reinforce positive habits.

Remember:

- **The goal is not perfection, but progress.** Embrace small wins and be patient with yourself. Some days will be easier than others, and that's okay.
- **Listen to your body and tailor practices to your needs.** Don't push yourself beyond your limits or force practices that don't resonate with you.
- **Most importantly, enjoy the journey!** Find joy in the small moments of awareness, the connection with your breath and body, and the positive impact these practices have on your overall well-being.

Congratulations on completing this 18-day exploration of Somatic Yoga! Remember, this is just the beginning. Continue to weave mindful movement and awareness into your daily life, cultivate your inner wisdom, and enjoy the journey towards a more empowered and present you.

Bonus Tip: Share your Somatic Yoga journey with others! Inspire your friends and family to explore mindful movement and create a supportive community that fosters well-being for all.

Day 19: Nourishing Your Body with Mindful Eating Strategies

As you continue your journey towards a healthy and mindful lifestyle, Day 19 focuses on **integrating mindful eating strategies** into your daily routine. Remember, nourishing your body with awareness and intention goes beyond calorie counting and restrictive diets. It's about cultivating a positive relationship with food and fueling your body with what it truly needs to thrive.

Setting the Stage:

- **Create a calm and distraction-free environment:** Turn off the TV, put away your phone, and choose a quiet place to enjoy your meal.
- **Engage in mindful breathing:** Take a few deep breaths before starting your meal to calm your mind and connect with your present state.

- **Express gratitude:** Acknowledge the effort put into growing and preparing your food. Offer a silent prayer or express appreciation to yourself or those who made your meal.

Mindful Eating Practices:

- **Ask yourself if you're truly hungry:** Before reaching for food, pause and ask yourself if physical hunger or emotional cues are driving your desire to eat. Consider alternative ways to address emotional needs, like exercise, journaling, or connecting with loved ones.
- **Eat slowly and savor each bite:** Put your fork down between bites, chew thoroughly, and pay attention to the taste, texture, and aroma of your food. This helps with digestion and allows you to truly enjoy your meal.

- **Honor your satiety cues:** Stop eating when you feel comfortably full, not stuffed. Pay attention to your body's signals and avoid overeating.
- **Choose nourishing foods:** Prioritize whole, unprocessed foods rich in nutrients. Include plenty of fruits, vegetables, whole grains, and lean protein in your diet.
- **Stay hydrated:** Water is essential for overall health and can help you feel fuller for longer. Aim to drink plenty of water throughout the day.

Beyond the Plate:

- **Practice mindful grocery shopping:** Plan your meals in advance and create a shopping list based on your nutritional needs. Avoid impulse purchases and stick to your list.
- **Read food labels:** Be aware of ingredients and portion sizes. Choose

foods with minimal added sugar, unhealthy fats, and artificial additives.

- **Cook more meals at home:** This allows you to control the ingredients and portion sizes of your food. Experiment with new recipes and discover healthy dishes you enjoy.
- **Mindful snacking:** Choose healthy snacks like fruits, vegetables, nuts, or yogurt when needed. Avoid mindless snacking while watching TV or working.

Remember:

- **Mindful eating is a journey, not a destination.** Be patient with yourself as you learn new habits and cultivate awareness around your food choices.
- **Celebrate small wins:** Every mindful bite and positive choice is a step towards a healthier relationship with food.

- **Don't deprive yourself:** Allow yourself occasional treats in moderation. Enjoying all foods in balance can prevent cravings and foster a positive food mindset.
- **Seek support:** Share your journey with friends, family, or a registered dietitian. Having someone to hold you accountable and offer guidance can be helpful.

As you move forward, remember that mindful eating is about nurturing your body with love and respect. By tuning into your inner wisdom and making conscious choices, you can fuel your well-being and pave the way for a healthier, happier you.

Bonus Tip: Practice mindful gratitude after your meals. Take a moment to appreciate the nourishment you've received, not just for the food itself, but for the entire process that brought it to your plate. This fosters a sense of connection and appreciation for your food.

Day 20: Rest & Reflect - Honoring Your Achievements and Looking Ahead

Congratulations! You've reached Day 20 of your Somatic Yoga journey. Take a moment to **rest, reflect, and celebrate your accomplishments**. This is a significant milestone, and you deserve to acknowledge the progress you've made.

Honoring Your Achievements:

- **Reflect on your starting point:** Remember where you were when you began this journey. What were your goals, motivations, and any existing challenges you faced?
- **Acknowledge your progress:** Take stock of what you've achieved. Did you notice improvements in your flexibility, strength, or overall well-being? Did you discover new insights about your body and mind? Did you cultivate

habits of mindful movement and awareness?

- **Be proud of yourself:** Regardless of how big or small you perceive your achievements, acknowledge your dedication and effort. Celebrate every step you've taken on this journey.

Reflecting on Your Journey:

- **What resonated most with you:** Consider the practices, poses, or aspects of the Somatic Yoga experience that you enjoyed the most. Did you find specific sequences particularly helpful? Did certain themes or principles resonate deeply with you?
- **Identify areas for further exploration:** Are there aspects of Somatic Yoga you'd like to delve deeper into, like specific poses, breathing techniques, or philosophical teachings? Perhaps you want to explore

other movement modalities that complement your practice.

- **Challenges and learnings:** Reflect on any challenges you faced and how you overcame them. What did you learn about yourself and your practice in the process? These learnings can become valuable tools for future growth.

Looking Ahead:

- **Setting intentions:** As you move forward, what do you want to prioritize in your practice? Do you want to focus on strengthening certain areas, cultivating deeper relaxation, or integrating mindfulness more fully into your daily life? Set clear intentions to guide your future exploration.
- **Creating a sustainable practice:** Reflect on what helped you stay consistent throughout this journey. Was it finding a specific time or space for

practice, connecting with a community, or simply enjoying the process itself? Identify factors that contributed to your success and incorporate them into your future plans.

- **Openness to growth:** Remember, your Somatic Yoga journey is ongoing. Keep exploring, learning, and evolving. Be open to new experiences, different teachers, and unexpected ways that this practice can continue to enrich your life.

Remember:

- Every journey is unique. Celebrate your own progress and avoid comparing yourself to others.
- Small, consistent steps lead to lasting change. Don't feel pressured to rush or do everything at once.

- Enjoy the process! Find joy in the movement, the exploration, and the connection with your body and mind.

Beyond Day 20:

As you conclude this specific challenge, remember that **Somatic Yoga is a philosophy and practice that extends beyond these 20 days.** Use the learnings, insights, and joy of movement as you continue on your path to well-being.

Here are some additional thoughts as you move forward:

- **Combine Somatic Yoga with other healthy habits:** Maintain a balanced diet, get enough sleep, and manage stress effectively for optimal well-being.
- **Listen to your body and modify as needed:** Every body is unique and has different needs. Don't push yourself

beyond your limits and always prioritize safety and mindful movement.

- **Be kind and compassionate to yourself:** This is a journey of exploration and self-discovery, not a competition. Celebrate your progress and be patient with yourself on challenging days.

Thank you for embarking on this journey with me! Wishing you continued joy, growth, and well-being as you continue your Somatic Yoga exploration and beyond.

Chapter 5

Bonus Week

Day 21-28: Exploring Advanced Somatic Yoga Practices - Deepening Your Journey

As you've completed the 20-day Somatic Yoga foundation, you're now ready to ** delve deeper** into more advanced practices and personalize your exploration based on your interests and goals. Remember, this is a continuous journey of self-discovery and mindful movement.

Exploring Different Areas:

- **Deepen your understanding of key principles:** Focus on specific aspects like breathwork, alignment, or proprioception to refine your practice and connect more deeply with your body's sensations.

- **Challenge yourself with more complex poses:** Gradually progress to more challenging poses like arm balances, inversions, or backbends, always prioritizing proper form and mindful transitions.
- **Explore variations and modifications:** Learn different ways to adapt poses to your unique needs and abilities, ensuring a safe and accessible practice.
- **Incorporate props effectively:** Utilize props like blocks, bolsters, straps, and chairs to enhance your alignment, deepen stretches, and support more challenging poses.
- **Focus on specific goals:** Whether you want to improve flexibility, build strength, or cultivate deeper relaxation, tailor your practice with poses and sequences that cater to your desired outcomes.

Resources for your Exploration:

- **Workshops and retreats:** Immerse yourself in deeper learning through workshops or retreats focused on specific aspects of Somatic Yoga.
- **Yoga books and articles:** Delve into books and articles by renowned Somatic Yoga teachers to gain deeper theoretical understanding and explore different perspectives.

Remember:

- **Safety first:** Always prioritize proper alignment and listen to your body's signals. Don't push yourself beyond your limits or force poses that cause pain.
- **Enjoy the process:** As you explore more advanced practices, remember to find joy in the movement, the exploration, and the connection with your inner wisdom.

- **Celebrate small wins:** Progress takes time and dedication. Acknowledge and celebrate your efforts, no matter how small they seem.
- **Be patient and kind to yourself:** There will be days when you feel challenged or frustrated. Be patient with yourself, learn from setbacks, and keep moving forward.

Here are some specific practices you can explore based on your interests:

- **For deeper relaxation:** Explore restorative yoga poses, supported inversions, and guided meditations specifically designed for Somatic Yoga.
- **For improved flexibility:** Focus on yin yoga sequences, dynamic stretches, and poses that target tight areas like the hips, hamstrings, and shoulders.
- **For increased strength:** Practice variations of Sun Salutations,

incorporate isometric holds in poses, and explore more challenging balancing postures.

- **For mindful breathwork:** Dedicate time to pranayama practices, explore different breathing techniques, and observe the connection between your breath and movement.

Remember, this is just a starting point. There are endless possibilities for exploration in the vast world of Somatic Yoga. Trust your intuition, experiment with different practices, and continue to cultivate a joyful and mindful journey towards your well-being goals.

Wishing you continued growth, discovery, and empowerment as you move forward on your Somatic Yoga path!

Conclusion

Your Lighter You Journey Continues!

Congratulations on completing this 28-day exploration of Somatic Yoga! You've embarked on a path of mindful movement, self-discovery, and connection with your inner wisdom. Remember, this is just the beginning of your **Lighter You journey**.

Reflecting on Your Transformation:

- **Embrace the shifts:** Take a moment to acknowledge the changes you've experienced. Do you feel more flexible, stronger, or calmer? Has your relationship with food improved? Have you gained new insights about your body and mind?
- **Celebrate your achievements:** Be proud of yourself for showing up, stepping outside your comfort zone, and exploring new ways to move and

connect with yourself. Every step forward is a victory!

- **Identify remaining challenges:** Are there areas where you still struggle or wish for improvement? Acknowledging these can help you continue setting meaningful goals for your ongoing journey.

Continuing Your Somatic Journey:

- **Integrate mindful practices:** Remember, Somatic Yoga isn't confined to the mat. Incorporate mindful movement and awareness into your daily life, whether through micro-stretches at your desk, mindful walking, or simply bringing intentional attention to your breath.
- **Personalize your exploration:** Choose practices that resonate with you and align with your goals. Whether you want to deepen relaxation, explore

advanced poses, or focus on specific areas of the body, cater your practice to your unique needs and desires.

- **Seek inspiration and support:** Continue learning from online resources, books, workshops, or even finding a local Somatic Yoga community. Sharing your journey with others can enhance your motivation and provide valuable support.

Remember:

- **Focus on progress, not perfection:** There will be good days and challenging days. Be patient with yourself, celebrate your progress, and learn from setbacks.
- **Listen to your body:** Always prioritize safety and well-being. Modify poses, take breaks, and rest when needed. This is your practice, and you get to set the pace.

- **Enjoy the process:** Find joy in the movement, the self-discovery, and the connection with your body and mind. Somatic Yoga is a lifelong journey, not a destination.

As you move forward, remember that you are lighter not just physically, but also mentally and emotionally. You've cultivated tools for stress management, self-awareness, and a deeper connection to your inner wisdom. Carry these tools with you as you continue your journey towards a healthier, happier, and lighter you!

Bonus Tip: Share your Somatic Yoga experience with others! Inspire your friends and family to explore mindful movement and create a ripple effect of well-being in your community.

Remember, I'm here to support you on your journey! As a large language model, I can't practice yoga myself, but I can offer information, resources, and encouragement as you continue your exploration.

Wishing you all the best on your continued journey towards a lighter and more empowered you!

Sample Somatic Yoga Sequences for Each Week

Here are some sample Somatic Yoga sequences for each week, focusing on different themes and incorporating variety while keeping the practice accessible for various levels:

Week 1: Introduction to Somatic Yoga:

- **Warm-up:** Gentle neck rolls, shoulder shrugs, arm circles, Cat-Cow pose, Downward-Facing Dog.
- **Standing poses:** Modified Warrior I, Warrior II, Triangle pose, Tree pose, Half Moon pose (optional).
- **Seated poses:** Seated Forward Fold, Seated Twist, Hero pose.
- **Supine poses:** Child's pose, Bridge pose, Supported Savasana.
- **Cool-down:** Gentle stretches, Child's pose, Savasana.

Week 2: Focus on Breath and Grounding:

- **Warm-up:** Breathwork exercises like alternate nostril breathing or box breathing, standing stretches emphasizing alignment.
- **Standing poses:** Warrior I with focused breath, Extended Side Angle pose, Mountain pose with conscious rooting.
- **Seated poses:** Seated Forward Fold with extended exhales, Supported Spinal Twists, Malasana pose (Garland pose).
- **Supine poses:** Supported Child's pose, Supine Figure-Four twist, Supported Savasana.
- **Cool-down:** Guided meditation focusing on the breath and sensations in the body.

Week 3: Exploring Flexibility and Balance:

- **Warm-up:** Warm-up flow with dynamic stretches like lunges and side bends, Cat-Cow with additional spinal awareness.
- **Standing poses:** Crescent Lunge with backbend variation, Triangle pose with deeper hip opening, Tree pose with eyes closed.
- **Seated poses:** Half Pigeon pose, Wide-Legged Forward Fold, Seated Forward Fold with forward bend variations.
- **Supine poses:** Happy Baby pose, Reclined Butterfly pose, Supported Bridge pose.
- **Cool-down:** Restorative postures like Supported Child's pose and Legs-Up-the-Wall pose.

Week 4: Building Strength and Stability:

- **Warm-up:** Sun Salutation variations with mindful transitions, Downward-Facing Dog with leg lifts.
- **Standing poses:** Warrior II with isometric holds, Chair pose with variations, Plank pose with modifications.
- **Seated poses:** Boat pose with variations, Chair pose with twist, Eagle pose (optional).
- **Supine poses:** Boat pose variation on elbows, Plank pose on forearms, Side Plank pose (optional).
- **Cool-down:** Supported Savasana with focus on grounding and releasing tension.

Remember:

- These are just samples, feel free to modify and adjust based on your needs and preferences.

- Always listen to your body and don't push yourself beyond your limits.
- Use props like blocks, bolsters, and straps to enhance your practice.
- Focus on mindful movement and breathwork throughout the sequences.
- Enjoy the exploration and celebrate your progress!

Creating a Home Yoga Practice: Your Personal Sanctuary

Building a home yoga practice can be incredibly rewarding, offering flexibility, self-care, and deep connection with your body and mind. Here are some tips to help you get started:

Setting the Stage:

- **Find your space:** Choose a clean, clutter-free area with enough room to move comfortably. Natural light and fresh air are bonuses!
- **Invest in a yoga mat:** This provides cushioning and grip, especially for floor poses.
- **Gather props (optional):** Blocks, blankets, bolsters, and straps can support various poses and modify for different levels.

- **Create a calming ambiance:** Use candles, aromatherapy, or calming music to set the mood.

Crafting Your Practice:

- **Define your goals:** Do you want to improve flexibility, build strength, reduce stress, or simply unwind? Tailor your practice accordingly.
- **Choose a style:** Vinyasa, Hatha, Yin, Restorative - explore different styles to find what resonates with you.
- **Find online resources:** Numerous websites and apps offer free and paid yoga classes for all levels. Consider Yoga Journal, DoYogaWithMe, or Glo.
- **Start small and be consistent:** Aim for 15-20 minutes a few times a week and gradually increase as you get comfortable.

- **Listen to your body:** Don't push yourself into pain. Modify poses as needed and respect your limitations.

Staying Motivated:

- **Track your progress:** Use a journal or app to note your practice dates, goals, and achievements.
- **Practice with a friend or join an online community:** Sharing your journey can be motivating and provide support.
- **Reward yourself:** Celebrate your milestones with a new yoga outfit or a relaxing spa day.
- **Focus on the joy of movement:** Remember, yoga is not about perfection but about connecting with your body and breath.
- **Be patient and persistent:** Building a consistent practice takes time and

dedication. Embrace the journey and enjoy the process!

Additional Tips:

- **Create a pre-yoga routine:** Light stretches, mindful breathing, and setting an intention can prepare your body and mind.
- **End with relaxation:** Savasana (corpse pose) or meditation can help you integrate the practice and ease back into your day.
- **Incorporate props effectively:** Utilize props to deepen stretches, improve alignment, and make poses accessible.
- **Don't compare yourself to others:** Everyone's body and practice are unique. Focus on your own journey and progress.
- **Explore yoga philosophy:** Reading or listening to podcasts about yoga can

deepen your understanding and appreciation for the practice.

Remember, your home yoga practice is a personal journey. Customize it to your needs, listen to your body, and most importantly, find joy in the movement and self-discovery!

Delicious and Mindful Recipes for Every Meal:

Breakfast:

- **Overnight Oats with Berries and Chia Seeds:** This recipe is perfect for meal prepping and provides sustained energy. Combine rolled oats, milk of your choice, chia seeds, and your favorite berries in a jar overnight. Enjoy cold or warmed up with a sprinkle of nuts and seeds.
- **Scrambled Tofu with Vegetables:** A protein-packed option for savory mornings. Scramble tofu with chopped vegetables like onions, peppers, and spinach. Add turmeric, nutritional yeast, and spices for extra flavor. Serve on whole-wheat toast or with avocado slices.
- **Green Smoothie Bowl:** Blend together spinach, banana, frozen mango, almond

milk, and protein powder for a creamy and nutritious smoothie bowl. Top with granola, chia seeds, and fresh fruit for added texture and flavor.

Lunch:

- **Lentil Soup with Whole-Wheat Bread:** This hearty soup is rich in protein and fiber. Simmer lentils with vegetables like carrots, celery, and tomatoes in a flavorful broth. Add herbs and spices like cumin, coriander, and paprika for a satisfying lunch.
- **Quinoa Salad with Roasted Vegetables:** A light and refreshing option. Roast your favorite vegetables like broccoli, sweet potatoes, and chickpeas. Combine with cooked quinoa, chopped cucumber, herbs, and a simple vinaigrette dressing.
- **Black Bean Burgers on Whole-Wheat Buns:** A delicious and

healthy alternative to beef burgers. Mash black beans with corn, bell peppers, and spices. Form into patties and pan-fry or bake until cooked through. Top with lettuce, tomato, and your favorite burger toppings.

Dinner:

- **Salmon with Roasted Asparagus and Quinoa:** A protein-rich and flavorful meal. Bake salmon seasoned with lemon, herbs, and spices. Roast asparagus with olive oil and salt. Serve with cooked quinoa for a complete meal.
- **Chicken Stir-Fry with Brown Rice:** A quick and easy option. Stir-fry chicken pieces with vegetables like broccoli, carrots, and bell peppers. Serve over brown rice with a homemade sauce made from soy sauce, ginger, garlic, and honey.

- **Vegetarian Chili with Cornbread:** A comforting and satisfying dish. Simmer kidney beans, black beans, and chopped vegetables in a tomato-based broth with spices like chili powder, cumin, and smoked paprika. Serve with cornbread for a complete meal.

Snacks:

- **Apple slices with almond butter:** A classic and healthy snack. Opt for natural almond butter without added sugar for the most nutritious option.
- **Carrot sticks with hummus:** A delicious and dippable snack rich in fiber and protein. Choose various colored carrots for added vitamins and minerals.
- **Greek yogurt with berries and granola:** A protein-packed and satisfying snack. Top Greek yogurt with your favorite berries and granola

for a balanced combination of carbohydrates, protein, and healthy fats.

Mindful Eating Tips:

- **Eat slowly and savor your food:** Pay attention to the taste, texture, and aroma of your food. Chew thoroughly and put your fork down between bites.
- **Distraction-free meals:** Turn off the TV and put away your phone while eating. Focus on the experience of enjoying your food.
- **Listen to your body:** Eat until you feel comfortably full, not stuffed. Stop when your body's hunger cues are satisfied.
- **Choose whole, unprocessed foods:** Opt for nutrient-rich options like fruits, vegetables, whole grains, and lean protein.

- **Cook more meals at home:** This allows you to control the ingredients and portion sizes of your food.
- **Hydrate throughout the day:** Water is essential for overall health and can help you feel fuller for longer.

Remember, mindful eating is not about restrictive diets, but about cultivating a healthy and positive relationship with food. Savor delicious, healthy meals while listening to your body's needs for a truly mindful and nourishing experience.

Journaling Prompts for Self-Reflection:

Exploring Yourself:

- What am I grateful for today? What are three specific things?
- What are my biggest accomplishments, big or small, this week/month/year?
- What is one fear I'm holding onto? How can I start facing it?
- What am I passionate about? How can I incorporate more of it into my life?
- What is one way I can express myself more authentically?
- What are my strengths and weaknesses? How can I leverage them both?
- Am I living in alignment with my values? If not, what changes can I make?
- What are my dreams and aspirations? What steps can I take towards achieving them?

- What is one thing I learned about myself today?

Relationships:

- How am I feeling about my relationships with friends, family, and/or romantic partners?
- Is there anyone I need to forgive, including myself?
- What am I giving and receiving in my relationships? Is it balanced?
- How can I communicate more effectively with those I care about?
- What kind of relationships do I want to cultivate in my life?
- How can I show more appreciation for the people in my life?
- What boundaries do I need to set in my relationships?
- Who inspires me, and why? How can I bring more of their qualities into my life?

- What is one way I can improve a specific relationship this week?

Mindset and Emotions:

- What are my biggest challenges right now? What are some positive ways to approach them?
- What negative thoughts or beliefs am I holding onto? How can I challenge them?
- Am I practicing gratitude regularly? How can I cultivate more joy in my life?
- What tools or practices can help me manage stress and anxiety?
- How can I show myself more compassion and self-love?
- What am I afraid of letting go of? Why, and how can I overcome that fear?
- What is one small act of self-care I can do today?

- How can I be more present and mindful in everyday moments?
- What am I avoiding? What would happen if I faced it head-on?

Remember:

- There are no right or wrong answers. Be honest and authentic with yourself.
- Write freely and without judgment. Allow your thoughts and feelings to flow onto the page.
- Don't overthink it! Some days, a few sentences are all you need.
- Be consistent. Try journaling for 10-15 minutes daily or weekly, whatever works for you.
- Review your entries regularly to track your progress and gain insights.
- Most importantly, enjoy the process of self-discovery!

Bonus:

- Use different prompts or create your own based on what's happening in your life.
- Experiment with different journaling styles, like bullet journaling, mind maps, or freewriting.
- Incorporate creative elements like drawings, quotes, or photos to enhance your experience.
- Share your journaling journey with a trusted friend or join a journaling community for support and inspiration.

I hope these prompts spark meaningful self-reflection!

Bonus

Video link for tutorials

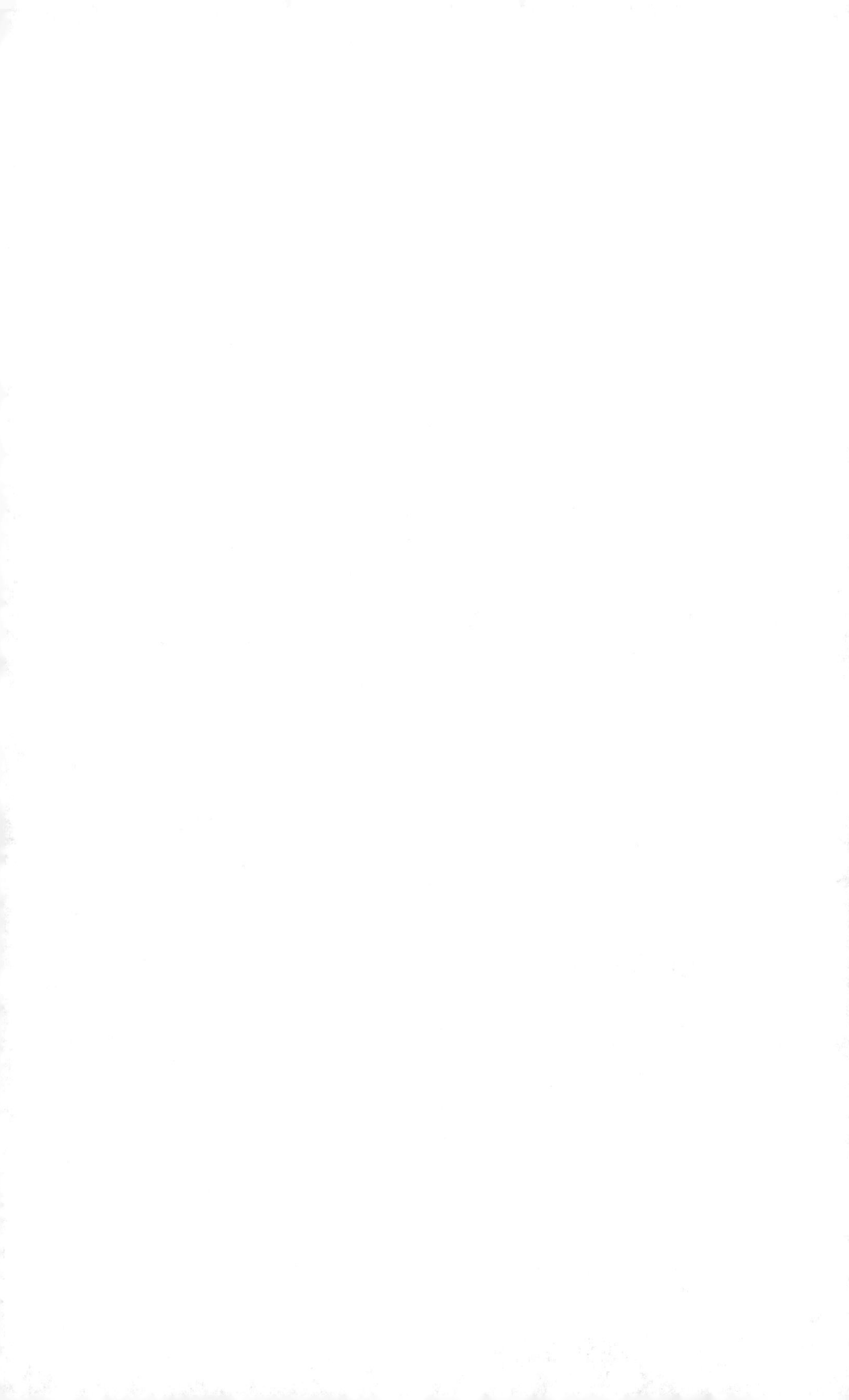

www.ingramcontent.com/pod-product-compliance
Lightning Source LLC
Chambersburg PA
CBHW050811260726
48660CB00004B/1374